"Dr. Jackie's book provides a holistic approach to help people cope with their daily pain. *The Mindfulness Solution to Pain* provides hope to anyone who is suffering and losing function as a result of constant pain."

> —Sol Stern, MD, chairman of Palliative Care at Halton Healthcare Services in Oakville, ON, Canada

"*The Mindfulness Solution to Pain* is a very practical and valuable addition to the toolbox of strategies for patients living with pain."

> —Roman D. Jovey, MD, past president of the Canadian Pain Society

"So often, chronic pain can be a life-destroying event that the medical world seems ill-equipped to manage. This is a wonderful guidebook for those who want strategies that do not simply make their pain better, but make themselves better with their pain."

> —Pam Squire, MD, assistant clinical professor at the University of British Columbia

"Chronic pain is common, disabling, and exhausting. Pain medications provide partial relief, but may not improve function or overall quality of life. What I like most about this book is that the authors embrace conventional approaches to pain management, but recognize that often this is not enough to allow pain sufferers to get on with their lives. Gardner-Nix and Costin-Hall provide an important alternative—mindfulness and meditation techniques that can revitalize the lives of those suffering with chronic pain. *The Mindfulness Solution to Pain* is presented with clarity and elegance, and I highly recommend this book to all chronic pain sufferers who need a boost to get their lives back on track."

> —Dwight Moulin, MD, Earl Russell Chair of Pain Management at the University of Western Ontario

the mindfulness solution to pain

Step-by-Step Techniques for Chronic Pain Management

Dr. Jackie Gardner-Nix
with Lucie Costin-Hall, MA

New Harbinger Publications, Inc.

Publisher's Note

Distributed in Canada by Raincoast Books

Copyright © 2009 by Jackie Gardner-Nix
       New Harbinger Publications, Inc.
       5674 Shattuck Avenue
       Oakland, CA 94609
       www.newharbinger.com

Cover design by Amy Shoup
Text design by Michele Waters
Acquired by Jess O'Brien
Edited by Kayla Sussell

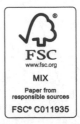

FSC
www.fsc.org
MIX
Paper from
responsible sources
FSC® C011935

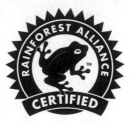

Library of Congress Cataloging-in-Publication Data

Gardner-Nix, Jackie.
  The mindfulness solution to pain : step-by-step techniques for chronic pain management / Jackie Gardner-Nix with Lucie Costin-Hall ; foreword by Jon Kabat-Zinn.
    p. cm.
  Includes bibliographical references.
  ISBN-13: 978-1-57224-581-5 (pbk. : alk. paper)
  ISBN-10: 1-57224-581-6 (pbk. : alk. paper) 1. Chronic pain--Alternative treatment. 2. Mindfulness-based cognitive therapy. I. Costin-Hall, Lucie. II. Title.
  RB127.G37 2008
  616'.0472--dc22

                          2008039793

15   14   13

10   9   8   7   6   5   4

contents

foreword

Jon Kabat-Zinn

All of us know on some level that pain is an inevitable part of the human condition, even if we sometimes shun that realization or pretend that we ourselves are immune to it. What is less well known is that there are many ways available to us to actually meet chronic or persistent pain and work with it, such that it does not inevitably have to lead to unending suffering and the complete erosion of a satisfying life. But when we are actually in the clutches of pain, whether it be primarily somatic or emotional (and it is invariably a mix of the two), and traditional medical approaches have not led to reliable relief, any way to go through the pain to an oasis of respite seems virtually inconceivable. In such moments, it is all too easy to fall into despair and depression.

It is for this reason that the book you have in your hands is so important. It could metaphorically and literally save your life and give it back to you, as so many of the people my colleagues and I have worked with in our mindfulness-based stress reduction clinic have actually told us over the years, and as you will hear from many of the people featured in this book. The systematic mindfulness practices offered here by Dr. Jackie Gardner-Nix and her colleague and former patient, Lucie Costin-Hall are based on their extensive clinical experience gathered over many years of working with people with very challenging chronic pain conditions. The authors offer a range of ways to discover for yourself that whatever you may be facing, it is indeed *workable* if you are willing to do a certain amount of interior exploring and adventuring and you are open to finding out how it might be possible to mobilize your own deep inner resources for learning, growing, healing, and transformation; resources available to all of us across our lifespan, but often so obscured or camouflaged that we hardly know they exist. This will be a part of the learning trajectory you embark upon here.

Often people with chronic pain conditions are told, once all the testing and diagnosing have been completed, that "You're going to have to learn to live with this." But sadly, that is often also the end of the story. There are few recommendations for *how* one goes about acquiring this learning, once all of the more traditional medical options have been used up. That is the purpose of this book. Moreover, there are few recommendations for how we can be supported in the process so that we don't feel so isolated and alone and, sometimes, even crazy and misunderstood. That is also the purpose of this book.

The Mindfulness Solution to Pain is a doorway into the universe of *mindfulness*, a particularly potent way of paying attention in your own life and of cultivating greater awareness, always starting from where you actually are and what you are actually experiencing. It is based on Dr. Gardner-Nix's many years of clinical experience teaching mindfulness to hundreds of people suffering from chronic pain conditions who were either not being helped by more traditional medical approaches, or were actually harmed by inappropriate attempts at medical treatment; it is also based on the firsthand experience of her former patient and now contributing author and colleague, Lucie Costin-Hall.

You might find yourself inwardly saying at this point, or even exclaiming aloud: "Paying attention? Awareness? I don't want to pay attention to my pain. I don't want to be *more* aware of it. More intimate with it. I want just the opposite. I want it to go away."

This is not an uncommon first reaction to hearing about mindfulness. And, of course, probably we would all want our pain and suffering just to magically go away, if only that were possible. But the amazing thing, which you can find out only by *practicing* mindfulness fairly regularly over time, is that paying attention in a particular way to the very sensations, emotions, and thoughts that together constitute the experience of pain—in the present moment and as nonjudgmentally as possible (which may be very judgmental a good deal of the time)—actually has within it the seeds of freedom from suffering. This is totally counterintuitive I know; nonetheless, it seems to be the case, as so many of our and Dr. Gardner-Nix's patients have discovered.

Approaching the pain itself, wherever it is most prominent in the body, with bare attention, open-heartedness, and alert interest even for very brief moments, if that is all that we can muster in any moment, can be profoundly healing, restorative, and illuminating. And if practiced over days, weeks, and months, potentially it can make a difference in the quality of your life for years and years going forward. What we are talking about is really befriending your experience at the level of the body and at the level of the mind and heart, and seeing what unfolds.

As the authors make clear, many of the practices in this book are based on our work at the Stress Reduction Clinic at the University of Massachusetts Medical School, work that has come to be known as MBSR or mindfulness-based stress reduction. Some of these practices are very similar to our approach, while others are either strong modifications, such as their particular approach to the body scan, or are uniquely Dr. Gardner-Nix's, such as the wonderful emphasis on pain drawings and their explications. Also, in some places, the authors suggest a distinction between *mindfulness* and *meditation* that I do not make. In my view, when we practice the formal meditations, we are cultivating the very same mindfulness that we are cultivating in daily life. That is why it is so useful and so powerful. Mindfulness is infinitely portable and, ultimately, is available in any and every waking moment. How you relate to life itself, unfolding moment by moment, however pleasant or unpleasant it may be in any moment, especially if you have a chronic pain condition, becomes the real meditation practice.

In MBSR, we emphasize that awareness and thinking are very different capacities. Both, of course, are extremely potent and valuable, but from the perspective of mindfulness, it is awareness that is healing, rather than mere thinking, however important and health-enhancing certain lines of thought and inquiry can be. Also, it is only awareness itself that can balance out all of our various inflammations of thought and the emotional agitations and distortions that accompany the frequent storms that blow through the mind, especially in the face of a chronic pain condition. Storms that along with the endless and often depressing stories we tell ourselves about our pain often wind up imprisoning us and severely limiting our options—even our hope because we become so attached to them as true when they may not be as true as we think they are.

From the perspective of mindfulness, nothing needs fixing. Nothing needs to be forced to stop, or change, or go away. With practice, mindful awareness can hold whatever is arising, whatever you are experiencing, and you will discover that things are always changing in ways that can clarify the learning you are experiencing and inform the various choices that are yours to make to enhance the quality of your life, as the authors frequently indicate. This capacity for mindful awareness is already your birthright, so you don't have to acquire it or do anything to achieve it. Rather, you need only become intimate with it through learning how to rest in awareness, even in the face of unpleasant sensations, thoughts, and emotions, even when they are very intense; in fact, especially when they are very intense. Sometimes we call this "dwelling in the domain of being" rather than getting caught up in the domain of doing and accomplishing, which is so often the habitual mode in which we face everything.

One of the most important elements of this work of mindfulness in regard to persistent pain is to bring awareness to intense body sensations as best you can, with an open and curious orientation, allowing yourself to hold these sensations in awareness, if only for very brief moments, if that is all you can manage. It is like dipping your toe in the water if you don't feel it is prudent to dive in all at once. By turning toward intense and unpleasant sensations in the body, even for a moment or two, and in the face of our own reluctance and aversion to do so, we are taking baby steps in befriending our body and reclaiming a full and nonadversarial relationship to it.

In this way, over time, we wind up learning a lot about our body sensations, discomfort, and pain, and we come to see that what we say to ourselves about them in the moment (like "I can't stand this any longer"), and what we feel emotionally (like "my life is ruined") are just our thoughts and emotions and they may not even be true. Our thoughts and emotions may actually compound the intensity and duration of our pain. When we become aware of them simply as thoughts and emotions, and feature the sensations themselves center-stage in the field of awareness, and learn to rest in awareness of the bare sensations, our entire relationship to them can change on its own. We may actually come to see and know deeply that we are not our pain—we are much bigger than it is—and that there are many different ways we can choose to be in relationship to intense sensations and even limitations that can help us to live and live well with things as they are in the only moment we ever get in which to live, which is this one.

Simple? Yes. Easy? No. But very much worth experimenting with in all the ways that this book suggests. For, ultimately, thinking and awareness inform and elevate each other and they can cooperate in giving your life back to you, and your body too, in ways that may allow you to befriend your body in spite of its limitations (whatever they might be in any given moment) and to appreciate your body in its fullness and learn to live inside it once again in peace, which is the deep inner meaning of the word *rehabilitation*. And mindfulness-based chronic pain management (MBCPM) is nothing if it is not an approach to full rehabilitation.

How mindfulness is defined and how to best cultivate it effectively in the face of pain and challenging life situations are issues that tend to sort themselves out over time with practice, as everybody makes the practice their own, modifies it as needed, and continues learning from their own experience, with the effective guidance of skilled mindfulness teachers. Then mindfulness becomes a skillful and kind *way of being*, rather than just a technique we invoke from time to time, or merely a concept that never gets out of the realm of thinking.

There is no single "right way" to cultivate mindfulness. Ultimately, with skillful help and guidance, like all of us, you will come to make the practice of mindfulness your own in unique and very creative ways. That is what this book is all about.

So here in this book, you have the entire curriculum of mindfulness-based chronic pain management as taught by Dr. Gardner-Nix and her colleagues. See if you can commit yourself to the adventure of taking on this program in its totality as if your life depended on it. Certainly, the quality of your life does; maybe the whole of it. What do you have to lose?

I wish you all the best on this adventure of a lifetime.

—Jon Kabat-Zinn
August, 2008/October 2008

acknowledgments

I would like to acknowledge Jon Kabat-Zinn and Saki Santorelli, without whose influence this book would never have been written: after twenty-two years in clinical medicine, they took the scales off my eyes. I would also like to acknowledge Jon Kabat-Zinn for reading the manuscript and offering suggestions which have enhanced this book so much: thank you. And to Kayla Sussell: you did a great job of editing the book; and Amy: we could not have hoped for better artwork for the cover: it was inspired. I also acknowledge my family, friends, and patients who have taught me so much; the phenomenal volunteers who have helped us with our mindfulness programs; the Ontario Telemedicine Network and hospital staff who enthusiastically made delivering our courses to distant communities possible; the summer students and medical students who have painstakingly analyzed our course data and with whom we have had such great discussions; and my two chiefs of the departments of anesthesia: Dr. Gil Faclier at Sunnybrook Health Sciences Center, and Dr. Patricia Houston at St. Michael's Hospital, who had the vision to allow us to establish our classes in mindfulness as part of our pain programs. And Lucie Costin-Hall, my contributing author: without her collaboration, encouragement, friendship, and enthusiasm I could never have taken what I now know and got it out there as effectively.

And finally, to my three daughters: Katherine, Victoria, and Elizabeth who each started their working lives by helping me in my medical office and aiding the summer students in tabulating our data. Thank you for coping with a medical mom and uncomplainingly sharing my attention with my patients in need.

—Jackie Gardner-Nix

I would like to thank everyone who presented me with difficulties in the past—for those challenges got me here. I would also like to thank my husband, Alex, and sons, Noel and Nick, for being such loyal supporters of my new life. And especially, I'd like to thank Dr. Jackie Gardner-Nix, whose ongoing friendship and expertise have guided me toward a better way of being.

—Lucie Costin-Hall

introduction

Pain is not just a "body" problem, it is a whole-systems problem.

—Jon Kabat-Zinn

- Stacey, a forty-five-year-old woman suffering from severe back pain, discovered her pain decreases whenever she goes to the family cottage on weekends. When she is there, she takes lower doses of her pain medications.

- Derek, thirty-seven, was on prescribed narcotics for pain, and on long-term disability for seven years as a result of four failed back surgeries. He then took courses in mindfulness and came to understand the mind-body connection. Nine months later he was jogging two miles a day. He has reduced his pain medications. He has also returned to the workforce.

- Cheryl, thirty-eight, was in a wheelchair, and on high doses of prescribed narcotics for severe chronic head pain after a neck surgery. She was also on oxygen because of the narcotics and had to be supervised by a paid attendant. Since taking courses in mindfulness, she has been able to keep her pain under control.

Her pain improved even further on divorcing her husband. Three years later, she's now out of her wheelchair, no longer on oxygen, on much lower doses of pain medication, and has returned to work.

Chronic pain, that is, pain lasting more than six months or beyond normal healing time, is usually much more difficult to treat than acute, short-term pain, and if you're suffering from chronic pain, we're sure you've noticed that physicians aren't exactly lining up to treat it. In particular, physicians who mainly specialize in the use of the really strong pain drugs, the opioids (narcotics), are constantly being sent the most difficult cases. Often, they seem to be considered the physicians of last resort. Our practice was full of what medical colleagues call their "heart sink" cases, a subset of the 30 percent of the Canadian general population who admit to chronic pain, a percentage that increases with age. New cases required at least a two-hour consultation just to get through the complexity of their histories and accounts of how many health care professionals they'd seen up to the present time.

the initial consultation

Emotions ran high in those initial consultations: anger at having to consult so many physicians, and at having their lives changed so radically by their disability, frustration at feeling they were not being taken seriously, and at looking so "normal" that others found them hard to believe. Frustration too at not "simply" being given the "strong" drugs that they thought would actually take their pain away and give them back their lives. What was it about health care professionals that we treated these patients' pain so badly? Didn't we believe them? Didn't we trust them with the strong drugs? They weren't looking to get high, they just wanted relief.

Frequently, tears were shed in our clinic, especially as we educated the patient and family about the fact that the drugs rarely got rid of their pain completely and would likely be only one of the strategies they might need to use for pain relief. For example, we once received a phone call from a man on the waiting list imploring us to call him immediately as it would take only ten minutes to explain his severe shoulder pain, an old injury, so that he could be given a prescription for the strong drug, methadone, that his physician was sure would take away his pain. Oh that it was that simple!

the bias against narcotics for pain

Many physicians are reluctant to prescribe strong opioids (narcotics) for pain except for patients who are dying. They fear their patients will become addicted to the medication but they may not realize that physical dependency differs from addiction. *Physical dependency* is the phenomenon of having to withdraw slowly from a drug, if stopping it, to avoid the unpleasant effects of withdrawal; *addiction* is the craving for a drug and going to any lengths to obtain it, despite the harm it does. Thankfully, this bias against using opioids even for severe pain is beginning to change, but the fact remains that fear of addiction keeps some of the most effective medications out of reach for many chronic pain patients. Doctors often refer these patients to pain specialists while subtly or not so subtly criticizing the specialist for prescribing anything stronger than a moderate painkiller.

Some doctors appear to believe that if the patient's pain is outside of the normal anatomical nerve distribution for where the abnormality is located, the patient must be malingering, or imagining the pain. Chronic pain patients are frequently given the message: "Your pain is all in your head." Funding agencies that handle disability claims tend to follow the opinions of such health care professionals, adding another layer of anger, frustration, and distress to the lives of those living with chronic pain. It's easy to see why physicians would rather fix broken legs than treat chronic pain patients.

dr. jackie's story: if it's okay for cancer pain, why not for noncancer pain?

I'd been interested in pain since medical school. During the 1980s, the Hospice movement was gathering momentum in the United Kingdom where I trained, bringing comfort at least to some of those dying of cancer. *Palliative care*, the care of the dying, was where I first learned my skills with the strong pain drugs and other ways of delivering comfort and pain relief. Gradually, throughout the late 1980s and into the 1990s, we saw a change in attitude toward pain, at least, by the innovators: it became okay to give the strong pain drugs not just to cancer patients but also to those who had severe noncancer pain. Some braver physicians and nurses, including me, even advocated that high doses were okay for the noncancer patients, if they didn't suffer side effects that canceled out the advantage of pain relief. But after working for a while with that as my attitude, I became not so impressed.

Dr. Jackie's Internship, 1979

"Why didn't we stop by that patient's bed?" I was asking a very authoritative nurse on one of my first ward rounds as a qualified doctor—actually a lowly intern, or houseman, as we were then called in the United Kingdom (UK). There was a saying that went like this: "Housemen were like mushrooms: kept in the dark, but every now and then, someone would open the door and throw shit on them." So I had to ask my question very respectfully. Otherwise, I might get a call at 4 A.M. from a nurse with a question that could have waited till after 8 A.M.

"That patient has terminal cancer," she answered in hushed tones. "There's nothing we can do for him. I suspect he's addicted to his pain medications. He asks for his pain medication when the pain is only just beginning to return." With that she turned her attention to the much more interesting story unfolding about the patient in the next bed, who clearly had something curable.

That was a pivotal moment for me. I thought, "Nothing we can do?" Surely our role ends only with death, and pain should be as much of a clinical challenge for us as any other medical condition. And why the scorn reserved for addicts, another medical condition worthy of our study, by so many who don't know what it's like to be in pain, or to be truly addicted? But I also couldn't accept that every person on strong pain drugs was to be regarded as an addict.

For many of my patients, the strong drugs were not getting them back to work, or even improving their function and quality of life, as much as I'd hoped. In most cases, muscles were weakened from underuse, so that painful joints and backs remained unsupported, and lifestyle habits had deteriorated. The pain drugs were just Band-Aids. They were useful if used as a means to help restrengthen and restore healthy lifestyles. Otherwise, they could even lead to reinjury by masking the warning pain that occurs from doing too much, too soon. Moreover, I learned that with prolonged use they even started to *cause* pain in some susceptible individuals. I also realized that for these patients their chronic pain issues were much deeper than giving them strong drugs could fix. With cancer patients the situation had been different.

As the tumors grew, we increased the medication, tolerated some sedation and other side effects, and eventually the patients died of their disease.

factors that influence pain

I was becoming aware that there were many factors that influenced the perception of pain. It was not all due to having a physical abnormality or malfunction.

Emotions and Pain

As the years went by, I followed the lives of the noncancer patients I had treated: those with low-back pain, joint pain, fibromyalgia, the abdominal pain of Crohn's disease and other diseases of the gut, headaches, facial pain, neuropathies, and on and on. I began to see a pattern emerge. I found that emotions did indeed play a part in the individual's perception of pain and possibly more: even the nerve irritation or inflammation at the site of the pain might change in response to emotions. The patients who had recently fallen in love, or who had left a difficult relationship and taken up another more meaningful one, would actually, in some cases, decrease their medication needs enormously. Yet the appearance of their Magnetic Resonance Images (MRIs) hadn't changed. The patients going on a vacation, whether to a country cottage or abroad, would frequently need less medication while away from home, only to see their medication requirements climb back up the minute the car got to the outskirts of the city again or the plane touched down on the tarmac.

Vivette's Pain Vacation

Vivette, a petite Caribbean woman, first began seeing me many years ago, when she had been in conflict with her rheumatologist for wanting too many painkillers for her rheumatoid arthritis. She had no drug plan and was too young for the seniors' plan so I suggested using a very small dose of methadone as it was so inexpensive. Thankfully, she did very well on it and was able to take just 5 mg, a small dose, every twelve hours for several years after, thus avoiding popping so many painkillers, which had lasted only for three hours anyway. And she was easily able to afford the medication.

Over the next few years she sometimes disappeared for months at a time and reappeared for an appointment several weeks after she should have run out of medication, if she had been taking the prescribed dose. She had always visited one of the Caribbean islands, staying with friends, usually for several months. She explained to me that when she was there, she suffered less pain, and lowered her dose. So it was not surprising that one day, when she was telling me that her pain had been worse lately, I asked why she had not considered moving back there for good. "After all," I said, "clearly the climate is good for your arthritis."

"It wouldn't work, Doctor" she told me. "The climate helps but that isn't it. If I moved there, my pain would be worse because I would take all my cares and responsibilities with me." And she went on to recount how her pain gradually increased during the plane ride back to Canada, and was present at its usual "Toronto" intensity the minute she stepped back inside her house.

I checked out Vivette's story with some other patients, and they really related to it. They too had stories of their pain receding when they got to the outskirts of Toronto on the way to the weekend cottage, only to be picked up again, like the dry cleaning, when they reentered the city limits.

One patient had been arrested by the police and charged, after they found several plastic bags of his opioid pills in his car when he'd been stopped in a police blitz to detect drunk drivers. They were convinced he must have been dealing drugs. It turned out he put the pills he didn't need to use into plastic bags when he was up at his trailer in the countryside, and had accumulated them over the summer. His medication needs went down when at the trailer, but he stockpiled for a rainy day; the day I might not be around to prescribe, I suppose.

Research has shown that anger affects how much pain we feel (Bruehl et al. 2002), and that it can even increase the doses of narcotics needed to reduce pain (Bruehl et al. 2003). The mother who gets chest pain after an argument with her adult son is truly suffering pain brought on by her emotion. We've known for years that emotions can cause physical symptoms. Phrases like "bored to death," "you make me sick," "paralyzed with fear," and, "she's a pain in the neck" are peppered throughout our language. I began to be aware of that when I was a palliative physician caring for cancer patients.

I saw that patients experiencing family arguments, for example, had their pain rise out of control and needed higher doses of medication, only to have the pain meds drop back to their original doses when the family crisis was over.

Life Trauma and Pain

But another pattern was also emerging. As I took detailed histories of my patients' lives, I began to understand why some people just don't heal after an injury from which most people would spend only a few weeks in pain, while healing. Most of the patients I saw had had very challenging childhoods and pasts. As for myself, I began to suffer a sort of secondary post-traumatic stress disorder from listening to them. I needed to brace myself before going into work each day to see another new patient and hear the usual heartrending story. During every consultation I felt as though I was crawling around inside the patient's brain with a flashlight looking for clues. And I think I became good at connecting the dots for them.

Their life experiences were generating chronic stress they didn't even recognize, stress that eventually caused their bodies to break down. I studied the psychological literature and found there was much to learn there relating to chronic pain, literature on body memories, and post-traumatic stress.

Genetics and Pain

In the field of genetics, a specific gene was discovered that makes some people more sensitive to pain than others (Zubieta et al. 2003). And if there's one gene described, there are likely to be more. But we also realized that not everyone who's had a challenging childhood ends up with a chronic stress response that predisposes them to illness later in life. Some people cope better than others and don't respond as profoundly to the same stressors. And the reason why they cope better might be found in their genetic makeup, as well as in some other factors involving, perhaps, their upbringing. A combination of genetics and the challenges of early life might combine to change a person's response to an injury. Genetics also plays a part in individual responses to pain medications, including the narcotics (Pasternak 2001).

dr. jackie's introduction to mindfulness and meditation

Back in 2001, in my drive to solve my patients' pain problems, I found myself in need of relief from all this intensity, and I also had my own personal stressors, which didn't help my tendency to have migraine headaches, a familial pain condition. So I took a course for health care professionals in the U.S. with Jon Kabat-Zinn to learn mindfulness-based stress reduction and meditation. It changed my outlook on life: I left Canadian soil a physician; I came back a person.

While there, I also recognized that the one place I'd seen people being mindful was in palliative care. When people knew they were dying, they were mindful. How sad that we come to notice what's going on in our present precious moments only when they are in short supply.

On my return to Canada, the first patient I sent off to do a course in mindfulness was Lucie Costin-Hall, who later helped me to write this book. She was at that time one of my chronic pain patients. A year later, with her pain under good control, and no longer my patient, she became my first volunteer when we established our classes in mindfulness and meditation for pain patients. She later trained in counseling and since then we have been on many speaking engagements together.

lucie's story

If someone had told me when I first met Dr. Jackie that I would be taking meditation courses to manage my pain I'd never have believed it. As a child growing up, I often heard my father, a physician, exclaim, "90 percent of the patients I see have problems that are all in their heads!" His implication was clear: if any of us children were ill, we were "imagining" it. Our illnesses were not "real."

Years later, I've come to realize that my father was only half right. There is a psychological link to all illness. That's because we're human. And it needn't be necessarily pathological. Where he erred was in thinking that the pain was not "real." In fact, emotions are triggered by thoughts that trigger chemical chain reactions in our bodies which, in turn, can cause our bodies to become ill. The illness is real. So is the pain.

When I first came to Dr. Jackie for treatment as a chronic pain patient, I was going through the single most challenging time of my life. After routine surgery, I had developed a devastating and rare complication that nearly cost me both my legs. Dr. Jackie explained that the debilitating chronic pain in my legs was due to nerve damage causing what is known as *neuropathic* pain. I was fortunate that this pain responded very well to an antiseizure medication usually given to epileptics, but which also can help settle damaged nerves. My pain subsided and then completely disappeared over a period of several months, and I felt extremely grateful for her skills and to the pharmacological manufacturer of the medication that worked so well for me.

After six surgeries in one year, I felt healthy enough to return to work as a writing professor at a university. But over the next year I became embroiled in political struggles: my year's absence from my teaching position appeared to me to have resulted in my peers not granting me tenure—a permanent position. During this time my father's health declined precipitously and he died. Then, I began to experience a pain in my ribs that my family doctor diagnosed as *shingles*, a nerve condition brought on by stress. Dr. Jackie suggested I take a mindfulness course to help me cope with my increased stress. Over the next half year I struggled with the course, but I found it difficult to concentrate.

I took a retirement package from the university, and announced my departure to my students. The day after I walked out of the university for the last time, I developed a debilitating pain in my neck. It was so bad that I could not get myself up from the floor. For the next two months I lay on the living room floor with my feet up on the coffee table. My only outings were to the mindfulness classes. I would lie on my mat in the corner of the room and meditate as others around me did yoga or walking or silent sitting meditation.

Dr. Jackie gave me some fairly strong pain medications; however, unlike the anticonvulsant I'd been taking for the neuropathic pain in my legs, they did nothing to relieve my pain. This pain persisted for weeks. I saw a neurosurgeon who ordered tests, only to be told, when he looked at my MRIs, that yes, there was a protrusion of the disk in my neck area, but it was no worse than many other people also had—with no pain. He could operate but he "wouldn't recommend it."

A friend suggested that I should read *Mindbody Prescription: Healing the Body, Healing the Pain* by John E. Sarno, MD (1998). "Oh great," I thought, "just like my dad who wouldn't allow you to feel sick without playing a head game on you." I refused to read it. I'd been fed that bunk all through my childhood. I was not about to that start again!

Three days later, another friend delivered the book to my house. "You've got to read this!" she implored. I thanked her for her kindness and put the book aside unread, thinking it was some "nonsense" some people wanted me to read. But later, flipping through the pages, I started to read one paragraph about the potential physical consequences of unconscious rage: "[T]he real pressures of everyday life accumulate in the mind, and the body creates pain, or some other physical symptom, as a distraction to prevent a violent emotional explosion" (1998, 12).

Something clicked. Yes, I certainly had good reason to feel rage. Rage at my father who never listened to me as a child. Rage at my workplace because my colleagues perhaps had been fearful that I would become a long-term liability. I had a lot of rage. It was, according to Dr. Sarno, the unfelt feelings associated with this rage that were causing my physical symptoms and, this is where my father got it wrong, my symptoms were real. I wasn't imagining my pain.

I read the whole book in a day, reflected on my anger, and then gave myself permission to visit my "unfelt emotions." Interestingly, the neck pain disappeared within two days. It was replaced, however, by the most excruciating anger and misery I have ever felt. My mind became a tsunami of emotions. I can remember thinking at one point that the physical pain in my neck was preferable to the anger, rage, and depression that replaced it.

And then after a week, just as suddenly as it had begun, the emotional storm subsided. It was not completely gone, mind you. It took years of mindfulness practice to completely accept the perceived harm done to me and to replace my anger with the intention of forgiveness. But the storm had passed and in its wake I felt a new peace. Since that day I have never experienced that pain again. I am so glad that I never went for the surgery.

In 2003, I went down to the U.S. to do the course with Jon Kabat-Zinn and Saki Santorelli, as Dr. Jackie had done. I had a background in TV and media and, on my return, I began helping Dr. Jackie to create the mindfulness CDs that are used in our workshops. Over time, I became increasingly committed to this new work and, eventually, I obtained a Masters in psychological counseling. In 2005, I changed from being a volunteer and started working with Dr. Jackie full-time to cofacilitate the courses. Currently, we are filming a documentary series on chronic pain for TV.

mindfulness-based chronic pain management courses

Courses for our pain sufferers offer an important intervention for their pain management: the chance to get out and meet others who are facing the same challenges, and by so doing, to feel less alone and shut-in and different. A chance to influence each others' lives, commit to weekly outings, and by examining our damaged lives, figure out what can be done, together. You will hear about some of their stories in this book, benefit from some of their insights, learn you are not alone in your suffering, and that your "class" is the readership of this book.

We modified the course to become as acceptable as possible to the typical patient we were referred. We were considerate of our patients' enormous limitations in committing to anything, especially weekly, and especially as different as this was from the usual procedures, surgeries, and drugs. But we made it clear, the course was not an "instead of," it was "in addition to" the usual avenues for many. We also made it clear that we were not insinuating that their pain was "all in their heads," or that they were in some way deficient psychologically compared to those who healed in the normal time span or those who did not have chronic illnesses.

No, we wanted them to see that their thoughts and emotions modified their pain experience: to be either intolerable or manageable. In becoming mindful they could become aware of the incredible links between mind and body. In doing so, life might open up for them to experience less disability and suffering. For many of the more than 2,000 patients who have taken our courses, it has.

Currently, we enroll chronic pain sufferers throughout Ontario for our twelve-week Mindfulness-Based Chronic Pain Management (MBCPM) course. And since Ontario is such a large Canadian province, we also offer classes via telemedicine to hospitals in the outlying areas.

In our telemedicine courses, patients living in rural sites attend their local hospital and join our onsite patients at our Toronto hospital location through the TV screen, so the mindfulness class is taken by patients simultaneously at two or three different sites and we can all see each other and have discussions and meditation as if we were in the same room.

understanding pain mindfully

We believe that running these courses gives us an enormous advantage in understanding you as a chronic pain sufferer, as we now spend so many hours in discussions and meditation in the company of chronic pain patients. Every week they allow us to see inside their minds and as we search around inside them with our theoretical flashlights, we are eager to learn whatever they can teach us, to understand the nature of pain, and to discover ways to manage it. Eager also, to use this knowledge to show you how to become mindful to better manage your enormously challenging problem of chronic pain and disability, in addition to what clinical medicine can offer you.

It may seem surprising how becoming more mindful changes the way a mind reacts to stress, often changing the pain experience, even when the pain is coming from a damaged place in the body. One of the first patients we had in class was a man in his early thirties with a history of four back surgeries. He had been out of the workforce for seven years and was on a moderate to high dose of narcotics and other pain medications. He had driven over an hour to get to class and was so skeptical during that first class that we didn't expect him to return. But he did the daily meditation as requested, and when we arrived the following week, he had the chairs already set up for class.

Over the next couple of years he had an emotionally bumpy ride as he went through some of the soul-searching he needed to do, but eventually he came off his pain medications and is now back in the workforce and enjoying family life. He still has pain but the pain is not running his life anymore.

Where Is the Pain Really Coming From?

The emotions likely affect how much inflammation and nerve irritation occur at the site of physical damage, so emotional stability contributes to a more manageable pain perception. When we read the research (Boden et al. 1990; Boos et al. 1995), which shows that abnormal findings can be seen in the MRI and CT (computed tomography) scans of the backs of people with no pain at all, and that disc herniations are just as common in those without back pain as in those with back pain, we begin to see that we were chasing the wrong diagnosis.

The neurologist who headed the first university pain clinic in which I worked in the late 1990s insisted that part of the initial workup should always be to find the diagnosis; but in those days, he really did mean find the nerve(s) that is (are) being pinched. It seems that, although finding that nerve(s) is important, the true diagnosis really involves asking: "And why is there still inflammation and/or irritation of the nerves at that site on a constant basis, over years not months, and occasionally causing such intense pain? Is the mind, while under chronic stress, and most likely sleep-deprived, enabling the constant pain messages to continue and also responsible for the poor healing, and if so, where does that response come from?"

We hope to show you in this book that this question makes sense, and that it doesn't mean that you, as a person living with chronic pain, are solely responsible for your inability to heal, or for having a chronic pain condition.

The Mind-Body Connection

Your mind and body are constantly undergoing chemical reactions taking place in millions of cells, completely responsible for every thought you have and action you do. Every human being is one big laboratory. In the kitchen, you can't prepare food without the ingredients and the cooking pots to create the chemical reactions—through heat, for example—to create the meal. Similarly, you can't move a muscle in your body without a cascade of chemical reactions happening inside you that result in that movement; starting with an incredibly fast message from your brain, which, in itself, is due to the chemical reactions your thoughts start. Your very thoughts and emotions are chemical reactions.

So changing your thoughts changes those chemical reactions, even triggering changes in your immune system, the system you use to fight infections, cancers, and repair your damaged tissues. Perhaps this information will start to open up for you the understanding that working to become more mindful, and training your mind to meditate, can truly influence the rest of your body. One influences the other: it is called "the mind-body connection." Doing this work may even influence your responses to your medication.

how to use this book

In this book we'll take you through your own personal journey in understanding your mind-body connection. We'll draw on stories of others' life experiences that may help you to navigate your own exciting yet uncertain journey through this practice called "mindfulness." But you will really need to do the work in this book daily, not just read about it; and not use it just like a fad diet for a few weeks. This work is life-changing. You've probably picked up this book wanting exactly that.

It's best to use the book as an addition to the interventions you may have been offered by your physicians and other health care professionals, unless you have exhausted all of those possibilities. Working through this book will give you a lot to think about and some thoughts and feelings that arise may be painful. If that happens, you should talk to your physician or therapist to help you through the rough spots, but it is likely to be important to address, not ignore, those painful feelings.

The meditations are important and should be done daily to get the full benefit from this work. With constant practice, you will note that your reactions to stressful events will become less intense and you may recover more quickly: these practices are good for mind *and* body.

We hope you are reading this book with enthusiasm and an open mind, but you may be reading it only because your physician, or a friend, or family member was looking for something to recommend after everything else has been tried and failed. Check yourself out to see whether you are waiting for any excuse to find this "does not apply to you." As has been demonstrated in the illness of depression, when you're in a bad space emotionally, the human mind tends to support its ongoing sadness by evaluating just about everything that comes up in a negative light. That probably happens when suffering from chronic pain too, especially when the pain is at its worst and you're sleep-deprived, as so many people with pain problems are.

To help motivate yourself, perhaps you could invite a family member to do the work in this book with you. In our courses, family members suffering from secondhand "chronic pain" are full participants; their chronic pain is analogous to the secondhand smoke in a home with a cigarette smoker.

Chapter 1 explains why it is important to see this work as truly affecting the healing processes in your body. Chapters 2 and 3 will get you started on the practice of mindfulness both formally and informally. We suggest you follow the instructions in those chapters for a couple of weeks before reading chapters 4 and 5, which will help with any challenges that may have arisen in those two weeks. Taking it one step at a time is important so as not to get overwhelmed. Feeling overwhelmed is a common concern in chronic pain sufferers.

It's a good idea to start a loose-leaf binder so you can write about your experiences as you go through this book, doing the exercises we give you to do, and plotting your course, as you change the quality of the rest of your life. Taking notes will not only help you do the work but will also give you a way of looking at your progress over the months and years to come.

In the appendix, we've included a questionnaire, a pain scale, and an exercise that you may want to do now, and repeat when you finish the book, and every six months, if you keep up your practice and can remember to do them, for a while after that. One questionnaire looks at your pain catastrophizing thoughts: how much do you ruminate, and whether you magnify your pain or feel helpless about it. The exercise is the diagram called the PRISM test that will help you to assess your level of suffering. Do the pain scale too, although, in fact, the intensity of your pain might not be the best measure of the quality of your life or how much you are suffering.

You might also want to read the book by Elaine Aron: *The Highly Sensitive Person: How to Thrive When the World Overwhelms You* (1996) and take her test to see whether the description of being a highly sensitive person fits you. If you are, that will help to explain why your health has suffered, as we will explain later.

Making the Commitment

Committing to doing this work will ultimately increase your understanding of how your body and mind work and interact, why you have chronic pain, and open up your life in a whole new way. But this is not a quick fix for your pain; it does take patience, and you're welcome to bring your skepticism with you, just not your brick wall! This work with your mind offers you a vital way to manage chronic pain and illness and, in fact, a way to maintain your health on a long-term basis. The most important part of opening this book is opening your mind at the same time, and making a commitment to do the work we describe. Then, be brave and turn on your flashlight!

Chapter 1

getting started on managing your pain: understanding why you have it

Meditation is not to escape from society, but to come back to ourselves and see what is going on. Once there is seeing, there must be acting. With mindfulness, we know what to do and what not to do to help.

—Thich Nhat Hanh

You might ask: "Why have I been in pain for years, and someone with a similar story was completely healed? Why can someone have a terrible accident, fractured pelvis, fractured limbs, ruptured spleen, the whole enchilada—and end up a few months later with no pain? But my pain, even from a lesser injury or a milder chronic illness, stayed on and on and on? Is it really something to do with how my mind affects my ability to heal and function, or not function, with pain?"

We know that the way you handle challenging life events—and reading this book and doing the work in it is a challenging event—also depends on the examples you were set by your parents or whomever reared you. As a deeply impressionable child, you watched and often subconsciously copied for the rest of your life, the behaviors that were modeled for you. If your parents were quitters, you're more likely to be a quitter too. Or you might have noted that they were quitters and already changed that mind-set for yourself.

the mind-body connection

You may have forgotten any knowledge of biology and chemistry that you ever studied a long time ago, so we'll try to make this simple. The human body, like all living organisms, is made up of chemicals. This may be a hard fact to absorb when nowadays so many people think of chemicals as "synthetic" and "bad," and natural substances such as those we buy in the health food stores as "good" and "safe." Physicians are always quelling their tendency to roll their eyes when they encounter that misconception. But to show you how drugs and meditation work we have to refer to chemistry.

The Chemistry of Thought

Hormones are chemicals (hence the sentence "There was chemistry between them" in steamy novels); enzymes are also chemicals; and the various elements we measure in blood tests are all chemicals that give us clues about how well various organs, such as the liver and kidneys, are functioning. *Neurotransmitters* are the chemicals in your nervous system, including your brain, that influence your moods, your emotions, your thought processes, and every function in your body.

When the chemicals are out of balance in your mind and body, you malfunction. That malfunction could lead to a tight or weak muscle, an acidic stomach, an abnormal heart rhythm, a poorly functioning liver or kidney, a depression, a panic attack or a migraine: it all depends on what the particular set of chemicals is and where the imbalance is located.

Interestingly, thought processes also work by changing the balance of chemicals, and so do drugs. Health care professionals try to restore your chemical imbalances to nearer normal balances with drugs. But in many situations and, probably, the earlier the better, you also can go a long way toward restoring normal chemical balances by changing your thought processes too. At first, this might not work as quickly as drugs do, although it probably is longer-lasting. Moreover, thought processes have fewer side effects.

It's intriguing that "mediCation," as a word, is so similar to the word "meditation." Perhaps the "C" is for chemical, and the "t" for thought. Which one would you rather use to get better, if you were given the choice and training?

Nature and Nurture

Why do the body and mind break down? We've long realized that chance is seldom a major part of the reason for a breakdown. Through taking thousands of detailed patient histories, reading the research literature, and seeing the remarkable outcomes patients experience from our courses, we have come to believe that illness, both mental and physical, and healing after injury or surgery are affected by both genetics (nature) and the experiences to which you've been exposed in life (nurture).

However, it isn't the severity of the challenging life events you encounter that affects how much your body gets sick in the future, but how negatively and intensely you reacted to those events; and how your parents or caregivers reacted. By showing you when you were a child how they, the adults, managed stressful events, they were a major influence on how you cope as an adult. Managing stress, which may have been very challenging when you were a child (the most impressionable time of your life) without good parental nurturing, apparently changes how you manage stress as an adult, even at the level of genetic material. Chronic stress leads to a poorer functioning immune system, the system that is crucial for body repair.

In David Suzuki's program, *The Nature of Things—Passion and Fury: Anger* shown on Canadian television (CBC), he described a study in chimpanzees, which showed that the teenage ape deprived of maternal attention when young is alright when life is routine, but becomes very stressed in adverse situations, especially when compared to maternally well-nurtured teenaged counterparts. Both morphine and antidepressants help the maternally deprived apes to cope better when facing challenges in teen and adult life. It is likely that those studies contribute to the understanding of addictions. But they also suggest that the quality of the parenting received in childhood is crucial in causing adults to be more or less vulnerable to the body malfunctioning later in life.

For example, you may have the genes in your genetic material to develop rheumatoid arthritis; but those genes might never be expressed in your body if it were not for certain events in your life that "activate" them. And those events may be multiple. *Psoriasis*, a skin disease that runs in families, for example, is known to cause itchy rashes to break out at times of stress, which could include a combination of several mild stressors, such as an emotional upset combined with sleep deprivation, and poor eating habits. Jon Kabat-Zinn and colleagues (1998) demonstrated that psoriasis sufferers, who were meditating when they received healing light therapy, had an increased rate of healing of their rashes when compared to a control group of psoriasis sufferers who received healing light therapy alone without meditating.

If you cope well with stress because during your childhood your caregivers showed you how to cope by example and teaching, or because you were born with a temperament that tends toward stoicism, you may never encounter a disease for which you have a genetic predisposition. But if events were very stressful in your early life or your parenting was deficient—and this isn't a blame game—this is just describing how it works, your stress system goes on high alert easily and frequently; and you may be more likely to develop an illness or disease or not heal well after surgery or an injury.

It's also helpful to understand that if you had inadequate or poor nurturing from your caregivers, it is likely that they, too, were poorly parented. Inadequate nurturing skills are handed down generation after generation unfortunately, until someone breaks the cycle. But you can't fix what you can't see. Mindfulness helps us to see.

the biology of stress

Emotional distress causes stress hormones to fire up: you may have heard of the fight-or-flight reflex. When that reflex response to stress happens, several processes in your body that are not essential for your immediate survival slow down and go on "hold." So, the processes of your gastrointestinal tract slow down (you may feel nauseous when upset), and your immune system also slows (you become more open to infection and you heal more slowly). But the body processes that can help you to survive are activated and go on high alert. For example, your heart beats faster because it is affected by the extra amount of adrenaline that is fired up to power your muscles (which tense up) to run from or fight the threat, and because you are on high alert, your sleep is disrupted.

Elaine Aron, in *The Highly Sensitive Person: How to Thrive When the World Overwhelms You* (1996), describes highly sensitive individuals, who tend to anticipate events strongly, also have more intense reactions to stressors and recover from stress more slowly. These characteristics appear in many of our chronic pain sufferers, and it may be reassuring to know that being highly sensitive may be partly caused by a genetic predisposition. For example, variants of a gene called the COMT gene have been described to account for differing sensitivities to physical pain (Zubietta et al. 2003). And a gene coding for a transporter protein for the neurotransmitter serotonin has been described, in which variants of the transporter protein, combined with early childhood stressors, predict the onset of depression by the person's mid-twenties.

Thus, if you are a highly sensitive individual, intense stressors in your early life are that much more disruptive to your whole mind-body system than someone born with the more stoical version of the COMT gene. Repeated fight-or-flight reactions to stress also can lead to a chronic state of stress, which you may not recognize because after living with chronic stress for some time, you may come to believe that is what it's like to feel normal.

The superwoman high achiever. For example, if your life fits the description of a high-achieving superwoman, you might not even know what it feels like to stop and take a break. You may have been trying to prove your worth since childhood. Perhaps your caregivers were particularly critical of you. Then, every muscle and nerve fiber in your body may have been set at high alert for years and your sleep may have been inadequate for months to years.

So when an injury occurs, the dramatic decrease in your functioning, combined with your diminished immune system function, your increased sleep deprivation, and your intense anxiety about being unable to keep going lead to the release of even more stress hormones. All of these factors then lead to even greater disability and pain than would normally be expected from your injury.

You might ask, "So why did I recover just fine when I had whiplash after a car accident when I was in my twenties?" The answer is that it's likely the younger body is more "forgiving" and capable of repair. With increasing life experiences layered on top of the very challenging ones encountered in your early life, your body is not as capable of bouncing back. The average age of pain sufferers attending our pain clinic and classes is forty-five.

The Connection Between Stress and Health

The simple messages are these: A lot of negative stress, especially in childhood, is bad for your health. *Chronic* (long-lasting) stress is bad for your long-term health. The more sensitive you are, which is partly programmed by your genetics, the more likely you are to react profoundly to stress with every cell in your body.

Good parenting, if you were lucky enough to get it, might have canceled out or reduced your high sensitivity and reactivity to stressful situations; thus teaching you how to respond to stress better is especially important for highly sensitive people. This, in turn, would have helped your body to become more resilient to life's challenges in your adult years too, even in stressful situations, by promoting better healing, restorative sleep patterns, and less likelihood of contracting a chronic illness or of never healing from a slipped disc.

Differences in health outcomes between siblings might be explained by genetics influencing whether you are highly sensitive or more stoical, but stressors involving parental nurturing may also have been different from one sibling's childhood to the next. Parenting styles might also have suited one sibling more than another. For example, high-achieving parents might have been well suited to the ambitious child, but might have been overwhelming for the sibling who was very sensitive to criticism.

Many of our parents were also born sensitive, had their own challenges in childhood, and did not have good role models in their parents. Therefore, they were not able to manage stress well themselves. They also might have self-medicated with alcohol, developed depression or another chronic mental or physical illness—so the cycle keeps going. Terrence Real, in his excellent book on male depression, *I Don't Want to Talk About It* (1997), describes this cycle in-depth and suggests ways to stop this kind of dysfunction from being passed down generation after generation. In our opinion, this has huge implications for health, in general.

Emotions and Pain

Finding the right drug(s) to set things right is not always possible when too many things have gone wrong with the body-mind connection, so your inner resources must be harnessed to arrive at the best possible outcome.

Persisting negative emotions, such as helplessness and hopelessness, anger or frustration, can keep you sick. Just as antibiotics can't work well to fight infection if your immune system is compromised, pain drugs don't work well if the emotional state of the sufferer is persistently negative. Anger has been shown to increase sensitivity to pain and decrease the positive response to pain medications (Bruehl et al. 2002; Bruehl et al. 2003). An inability to forgive has been linked to an increased likelihood of suffering low-back pain (Carson et al. 2005).

A recent research paper that surveyed the literature going back to the early 1980s showed that psychological interventions for chronic pain conditions didn't just help people cope better, they also decreased pain (Hoffman et al. 2007). One huge study reported in the highly respected publication *The Lancet* in 2004, demonstrated that anger, depression, anxiety, lack of social support, and chronic stress all contributed to the likelihood of having a heart attack on a par with the physical stressors of smoking, obesity, high blood pressure, and high cholesterol (Rosengren et al. 2004).

Epigenetics. A newly emerging field called *epigenetics* studies what factors influence genes being expressed during a lifetime. (It takes the expression of certain genes to do anything in your body, including healing.) Often various stressors, both emotional and physical, can lead to genes becoming expressed. You might carry a gene or set of genes to develop a certain disease and never develop that condition if those genes are never expressed.

So in this book, we hope to help you through training in mindfulness to become much more aware of the roots of your emotions, of the ways your thoughts work, of why your body and your mind have been functioning the way they have been, which is likely not the way you want them to function. Mindfulness increases the awareness of the mind-body connection, so as you bring greater mindfulness to your experiences, even the most unpleasant ones, you may find yourself dealing with your chronic pain very differently. We begin at the beginning, by learning how to cultivate greater mindfulness, a way of being in relationship to your experience that you may have been familiar with only in your childhood.

Chapter 2

mindfulness: what is it?

getting acquainted with your inner resources (1)

You can see a lot by just observing.

—Yogi Berra

In this chapter we're going to describe what mindfulness is and show you how mindfulness and pain are linked. We'll also get you started on practicing mindfulness.

Mindfulness is the awareness that arises when we pay attention to what is happening in the present moment, nonjudgmentally; right in the here and now. Whether an experience is pleasant or unpleasant in any given moment, whether it is mundane or exotic, whether it involves our own thoughts and feelings or what is going on outside of ourselves, in the environment around us, mindfulness is being aware of what is unfolding inwardly and outwardly moment by moment. It is awareness itself, capable of holding and discerning any sensation, thought or emotion, as it is, without adornment or coloration, and especially without judging it as good or bad, desirable or undesirable. Mindfulness accords equal attention and value to what is happening in each moment of your life, whether it is an experience which you would normally have judged to be good, bad or neutral. Learning how to inhabit your own capacity for awareness can be profoundly transformative and liberating.

taking mindfulness with you on vacation

Think back to when you last went on vacation. Was your mind already ahead of you? Did you treat the journey as an inconvenient experience in getting there, and not as part of the experience to be savored? When you arrived, were you already planning the trip back home? And did your physical pain increase as you anticipated the challenges you would face on your return journey? Like most people, you've probably done this.

Yet you do see the value of having meaningful experiences while traveling: Why else would you journey far from home to experience the scenic wonders of the Grand Canyon, the majesty of Buckingham Palace, the splendor of the mountains of the Rockies or the Alps? But rather than standing there just looking, taking it all in and feeling the full impact in those moments, and possibly barely noticing your pain, were you reaching for the camera or the camcorder? And by doing that were you delaying yet again the precious moments of actually having the experience, until you saw them later on celluloid? Why is it that we set a higher value on storing experiences rather than experiencing them at the time they are happening? And that we hardly even notice what we consider to be mundane?

reclaiming mindfulness as an adult: not when it's too late

Mindfulness is often practiced intensely by one segment of our population: those who are dying. For many whose days are numbered, mindfulness returns and they begin to savor all of their moments, particularly if they have good symptom control. They even appreciate the mundane.

We remember one man who was dying of cancer, who had been mentally challenged his entire life. He lay in a hospital bed set up in his living room at home, and was cared for by a loving brother who happened to be an emergency room physician in the United States, who had taken a leave of absence to tend to his brother in his dying days. The dying man was one of the rare people we'd encountered who gave off a feeling of having always been in touch with the present moment. With skillful use of pain medications we were able to keep him comfortable. During his last twenty-four hours he was absorbed in listening to the birds singing outside his window, and identifying them with pleasure. For our team and his brother that was what good palliative care was all about.

Another woman, currently in her fifties, who has survived for five magical years after having been diagnosed with advanced ovarian cancer, is working her way through a list she made when she was in treatment. Her list names all the experiences she was determined to have if her life was to be spared. Today, she savors every moment and radiates joy. It's a pleasure to be in her company.

Reading this book can afford you a chance to reclaim living in the only moment you will ever have: this one. Why not take the opportunity, rather than run the risk of realizing at some point that somehow you may have missed large swaths of life while it was passing you by, that you were and maybe are only half noticing what's going on all around you and within you. This moment we call now may be your best and perhaps only chance to ensure that you are living life fully while you have the chance. But notice if you find yourself thinking at this point that this may not be possible in your case because of how miserable your life is due to your pain. Many of our patients felt exactly the same before launching themselves into the practice of mindfulness.

mindfulness during difficult times

Being mindful is not just paying attention to positive experiences, but also to the neutral and the negative ones. As a society, we tend to avoid paying attention to negative experiences and emotions and even run from them, depending on their intensity and our own tolerance for distress. However, avoidance of feeling the more difficult emotions can prolong their power over you and your health. Conversely, attending to these experiences and feeling the emotional pain they cause, even if you can only allow yourself to feel that intensity of suffering for a few brief moments, can shorten recovery from that pain and lower the impact on your bodily systems.

Learning to live from moment to moment is actually reassuring. The intensity of the sadness or grief you allow yourself to experience in mindfulness practice is always tempered by the knowledge that "this too shall pass."

When you make a point of noting your emotions from time to time during your day, you may be amazed by how much your feelings can change.

For the next week, a good start for practicing mindfulness will be to note, nonjudgmentally, as an observer, what is happening in the moments when your pain is worse, and what is happening when your pain has lessened and you feel better. Write down the events and look at what you wrote at the end of the week. But don't look only for movement-related pain changes; look at the situations that are taking place in your family or at work (if you still work), and at what sort of a night's sleep you had. Does your pain ramp up when you are on the phone with a difficult relative, or when you've had a stressful car ride, or when you read something bad in the newspaper?

Elena's Insight

Elena approached me at the end of the Saturday maintenance mindfulness class, looking worried. She'd been trained in our classes a couple of years before, and had been very stable on strong opioid medications over the last four years for her painful back, on which she'd had surgery in the past. But she told me that over the last few weeks, it had felt as though her medications weren't working as well as they had been. She was concerned, even frightened, that they were no longer going to give her relief.

There had been no trauma that had started this pain exacerbation. I asked her what had happened in her family life around the time the pain had increased. Her brow cleared as she made the connection—and she remembered to strengthen her mindfulness practice! Her husband had started drinking again and she hadn't made the connection that she'd been feeling extremely anxious that he might be reverting to his old drinking problems.

She left with the resolve to share this with him. He was a caring man, and was likely to watch his drinking, especially if it affected his wife's health. At subsequent classes her pain was back under control.

Attitudes Associated with Mindfulness

Attitudes can become habits which are learned from our exposure to the challenges of life, to others whom we copied, and perhaps due to genetics.

But if they have become destructive, with mindfulness practice helping you to become more fully aware, they can be noted and acknowledged as harmful to yourself. That becomes the first step to changing, as it becomes harder to continue to live with such destructive habits once you see them. Just seeing them clearly is the first step by which they can change.

Judging

In addition to noticing the relationships between your pain and whatever else is going on in your life, you might notice how much you judge situations and people. *Judgments* are made when you label experiences as either good or bad, negative or positive. Judging good or bad can become fast and automatic, but it is really a type of mental shorthand which substitutes for observing and describing the experience more fully, which perhaps might have lead to a different feeling and emotion about it.

You may be surprised at how many times you find yourself judging situations or yourself, no matter how much of a commitment you make to taking a more non-judgmental stance toward your experience. This is a natural part of the practice of mindfulness, so there is no need to judge the judging. Through the practice of mindfulness, moment by moment, you may come to see that tension is created in the body just by how much you react when you dislike something that is already unfolding as part of your experience. If you mindfully note the connections in this chain of events where a judgment or a thought leads to a reactive emotion, which leads to a muscle contraction and, therefore, to tension in the body, you will be in a much better position to free yourself from this habitual pattern simply by bringing awareness to it.

It can feel so liberating to look at people and situations and not constantly judge them. You might ask: "But how can I not remember the past hurts and disappointments that make me tense up? What choice do I really have?" Being nonjudgmental may seem an unattainable goal to you. However, the following fable may help you to better understand how judging events can be a misleading and ineffective way of dealing with reality.

The Farmer and His Horse

Many years ago, there was a farmer who owned a horse. This horse was the farmer's prize possession because he was very important to the running of the farm. One day the door of the barn was accidentally left unbolted and the horse fled the barn and disappeared into the nearby forest. "This is a calamity," the farmer's neighbors groaned. They knew that without his horse the farmer could not manage his farm. The farmer simply said, "Perhaps."

The next day, the horse, leading a herd of wild horses behind him, returned to the barn. All the neighbors exclaimed, "You are a very lucky man indeed! Now you have many horses to help you with your tasks." To which the farmer replied, "Perhaps."

Soon after, the farmer's only son was breaking in one of the wild horses when he was violently thrown to the ground and broke his leg. "This is terrible," moaned the neighbors. "Without the help of your son you will lose your farm," to which the farmer replied once again, "Perhaps."

The son was taken to the hospital for his broken leg, and in the Emergency Room he met a lovely nurse, whom he started to date. The neighbors exclaimed, "How wonderful that fate brought them together like this," to which the farmer replied, "Perhaps."

This fable can go on and on with many twists and turns, with each disaster turning into a victory, and every victory leading to a defeat. Perhaps you could be more like the farmer and remain more open and neutral about the events that arise in your life. You are aware of what your feelings are but, ultimately, you become mindful about the draining of your emotional energy by investing in those feelings. Maybe, like the farmer in the fable, you become aware that life's negatives sometimes turn into positives, and things that seem positive may not always turn out to be so.

After a few months or even weeks of mindfulness practice whenever you feel yourself starting to judge somebody or something, you may find it will become more natural for you to just to note how you feel, and then to describe what is happening nonjudgmentally. By doing this, you open yourself to the possibility that life is too full of unforeseen opportunities to waste your time investing in negative emotions for long.

Beginner's Mind

Approaching life with more of an observant and neutral attitude can be described as reverting to beginner's mind. The characteristics of *beginner's mind* are a tendency not to prejudge as much as you may have done previously, not to bring your past experiences into your current evaluations as intensely as you may have done before, and not to anticipate the negatives.

As a chronic pain sufferer, you are likely to be more highly sensitive to life's challenges than others, quick to anticipate and react to them, and quick to feel stressed. Your body's stress response, summoned over and over again, reduces healing. And although it might temporarily take your mind off your pain, more often than not, it's as though the pain goes on hold, only to return more intensely after the stress has passed. Acquiring the gift of beginner's mind through practice will result in anticipating negative events less frequently and less intensely. Your mind and body will become calmer and experience lower levels of stress hormones circulating as your practice deepens. Healing will increase, inflammation flare-ups will be reduced, and pain exacerbations may become less frequent.

Trust

It's worth starting to practice these attitudes right now, and if your first instinct is to say, "My responses are too ingrained now for me to act in new ways," you might be surprised at what will happen once you are aware of your "usual way" and can see how damaging it can be. Have trust that, with your increasing awareness, change may unfold on its own, taking both your mind and your body in new directions. Adults, even seniors, often start learning a musical instrument for the first time in their lives with all the agility the brain needs to do that. Many seniors take up the complicated card game of bridge and do well. They "install" and train new brain pathways every time they learn something new; and it becomes easier as they practice. You can do this too in the practice of mindfulness.

Patience

Throughout your learning of mindfulness and the formal practice of meditation you will need patience and humility. Mindfully becoming aware of old destructive habits will bring about change simply through your increased awareness but it will take time. Good things are worth working and waiting for, and increased happiness is a commonly reported result along the way. Trust that this process is within your abilities as your awareness and discernment increase, and don't shoot for the stars, at least not too soon. Have patience, and especially be gentle with yourself if you are starting to increase your exercise or move beyond your usual routines, as you mindfully look beyond what you set as your restrictions a long time ago.

One common fear when you try something new is that of failing. For example, if you decide to go to a movie theater for the first time in years, make it a slow, mindful experience. If you find yourself needing to leave the theater halfway through the movie due to pain, acknowledge your pain mindfully, including any negative emotion like disappointment, which is likely to come up. Be patient with yourself, congratulate yourself for doing even that much, and know that you may be able to stay longer the next time you go. It may take years, but becoming mindful and aware will bring about change.

Other attitudes like acceptance and letting go are also characteristics of mindfulness, but we will look at those later in the book. For now, let's move onto a formal practice of mindfulness: meditation, which is dealt with in the next chapter.

Chapter 3

meditation 101:

getting acquainted with your inner resources (2)

The complex is difficult to understand.
The simple, even more so.

—Anonymous

In this chapter you'll be learning how to meditate. We'll cover what meditation is, what positions to adopt to practice it, and we'll give you some guidelines.

what is meditation?

The formal practice of *meditation* involves intentionally setting aside a specific period, (or periods) in your day to systematically cultivate mindfulness by focusing your attention moment by moment on some particular aspect of your experience, and actively noting when your mind wanders—as it always will— and then bringing it back to the focus. The most convenient and important objects of attention to cultivate are sensations in the body, thoughts and emotions, and other aspects of sensory experience, such as hearing, seeing, touching, tasting, etc. Andrew Weil on his CD, "Meditation for Optimal Health" refers to it as "directed concentration (see recommended reading)." He uses the analogy of a focused beam of light to describe the focusing of the mind in meditation. During meditation, the thoughts jostling for your attention are left at the outskirts of your consciousness as you use the art of focusing on one thing, such as your breathing or a candle flame, to develop what is sometimes called "bare" attention.

In our classes, we usually use what Jon Kabat-Zinn in his courses and his book *Full Catastrophe Living* (1991) teaches; that is, using the breath as the basic focus. Breathing is accessible to all, and only a few people have reported that using their breath as a focus isn't comfortable for them, such as in those who have emphysema, asthma, or allergies.

Noting when your mind wanders, which inevitably happens every few breaths, and being nonjudgmental while bringing your mind back to focusing—without feeling frustration or impatience—over and over again, is therapeutic in itself. It allows you to observe when you're being hard on yourself and to practice, over and over again, being less judgmental of yourself. Moreover, it is actually quite an alert state to be in.

Formal practice is the act of establishing yourself in a particular body posture for a period of time for the purpose of systematically cultivating moment-to-moment non-judgmental awareness. We sometimes call this *formal meditation practice*. It is an intentional giving of yourself over to the domain of being for a while, and letting go of all the doing we are consumed with so much of the time. It contributes to recovering and reinforcing the sense that you are a human "being" rather than merely a human "doing." *Informal mindfulness practice* is allowing every aspect of your day to become part of your meditation practice, so that you are more openheartedly present and less reactive and judgmental in the ongoing activities of daily living, whatever they may be, alone and with others, under pleasant or unpleasant conditions, and with whatever may be going on inwardly in terms of your body sensations, emotions, and thoughts.

Meditation vs. Relaxation

Meditation and relaxation are often confused. However, there are basic differences between using relaxation therapy and meditating. The goal of relaxation therapy is to almost fall asleep, whereas the goal of meditation is to "fall awake"; that is, to become more aware, more conscious of your inner self. Relaxation tends to be the unfocused wandering of the mind and reducing the tension in the muscles of the body. Interestingly, the meditative focused state usually results in the muscles relaxing and, as you finish a formal meditation, you may look as though you are coming out from under a state of sedation. But unlike recovering from a dose of Valium (diazepam), your mind will get going again very much faster.

Physical Benefits of Meditation

It is being increasingly recognized there are many benefits to meditation. Research has shown that there are positive effects on the immune system (Kabat-Zinn et al. 1998; Davidson et al. 2003), just as there are in the deeper stages of sleep, which many chronic pain patients do not get or get too little of. Also, with regular practice, meditators report they feel their lives are less disrupted by challenging events and that they recover more quickly from such events (Goleman and Schwartz 1979). Because the body and mind are linked, this means that the immune system, the gastrointestinal tract, and many other systems are less likely to be disrupted when challenging events occur.

Interestingly, many of our regular meditators report they feel their pain medication works more effectively after meditating. They also report that if they suddenly stop meditating regularly, for example, on a vacation when they couldn't find a quiet moment to practice, they went into a state of withdrawal marked by agitation and restlessness similar to the withdrawal symptoms they experienced when they suddenly stop using a sedative or narcotic drug. In our opinion, this demonstrates a similarity between the chemical effects of meditation and medication on the mind and body.

Starting to Practice Meditation

Timing. Choose a time and place where you are not likely to be interrupted. This is the start of committing to a daily practice. Decide that if the phone rings, you will not answer it. Most importantly, choose a time when your physical and/or emotional pain is not at its most intense. If you are on pain medications that do not cloud your mind, you might time your meditation to take place at the same time that your pain medication works most effectively.

Duration. Just as you would find it best not to overdo it the first day at the gym, in case you might hurt for the next few days and would never go back to the gym again, it's best to set a reasonable goal for meditation too. Start by setting a timer for only five minutes, or even one or two minutes, if you think five will be too much for you. Eventually, over time you can increase your meditative time to twenty to thirty minutes; in fact, these are the most popular durations for most of our patients. It may feel strange and even boring at first, but in time, you'll come to look forward to your daily meditation.

Clothing and positioning. Wear loose, comfortable clothing, and choose warm clothing if you are likely to get cold while staying still for this period of time. Assume a comfortable position when doing meditation; preferably with your eyes gently closed. If you are completely able-bodied, we ask you to sit upright in a dignified posture on a chair. Sit a little bit forward from the back of the chair, legs uncrossed with both feet firmly on the floor, and hands gently resting on your lap.

You must try to sit so as to have no points of pressure anywhere in your body because this causes compression of the blood supply to the nerves, which is the reason that limbs sometimes fall asleep. Sitting in this dignified posture allows the air and blood in your body to circulate freely. Some people find it more comfortable to have their feet raised a little from the floor on a footrest: turning a chair upside down in front of you to rest your legs on might work best.

If you prefer and are able, you could try sitting in a lotus position (cross-legged) either directly on the floor or on a cushion or low bench on the floor, legs crossed and with your back straight. Or you might meditate lying down, symmetrically, if your pain condition permits. Lying down on the floor and raising their legs to rest on a chair seat is a popular position for our back pain sufferers.

However, if none of these positions is comfortable for you, find and create your own customized position. Meditation can be done from any position.

What to do with pain and discomfort during meditation. In the process of the meditation, you may find your mind going directly to your pain, and you might notice your pain increasing. If this starts to happen, note your emotions. The pain exacerbation is usually due to fear, particularly the fear of having nothing else to distract you. You may note what you say to yourself in that moment, such as "I can't stand this pain" triggers adverse emotions. Becoming aware of this self-defeating tendency by simply bringing awareness to it may allow you to peel away the components that make up your suffering pain experience, like taking away the layers of an onion. Is it possible to glimpse the bare sensation of pain, unembellished by thought and emotion? Is your awareness of the pain "in pain"? Just for a moment can you be present with the bare sensation of your pain, sort of like dipping your toe in the water when you don't want to plunge in because the water may be freezing cold, and therefore too distressing? And in that glimpse, can you see that you are not your physical pain, that you are much bigger than it is?

If you feel you must move to relieve your discomfort, bring your attention to your pain fully first and just "sit" with the awareness gently for a few moments; then, if you need to shift, do so. If you have an itch or an urge to drink water because your mouth feels dry, just observe the experience without automatically scratching or drinking. If you find that really intolerable at first, give yourself a break and scratch or drink.

Focusing on your breath. When you are in position, begin by observing your breath, at the nostrils, the chest, the mouth, or the abdomen but without changing your breathing in any way. This is not deep breathing. You can read the five-minute meditation guide below to see how to manage your thoughts while doing this, as thoughts inevitably will flow into your consciousness and try to take center stage as you settle your mind on your breathing.

Five-Minute Meditation

Choosing to spend five minutes in meditation
Just taking a few minutes out of the day
To fall awake
Going to the breath
Focusing on it
Perhaps at the nostrils
Or at the mouth
Or at the chest
Or at the abdomen
Whatever feels right for you
And not changing the breath in any way
Just using it as a focus

Breathing
Noticing when your mind wanders
And without frustration, nonjudgmentally
Just bringing it back to the breath
Focusing over and over again
On the breath
Being with this moment
And this moment
And the next

Living in these moments
In the here and now
Not thinking of the past
Not thinking of the future
Just being in the present

Creating your own center
For a few moments
Focusing on these breaths
Taking this time
Time for yourself

Tuning in perhaps
To any feelings or sensations
Within your body
And just noting
How they change, when you become focused
Focusing on your breath
The life force that goes to every part of your body
Breathing
Acknowledging being

And as these few precious moments
Come to an end
As you resurface back
Into the doing part of your life
Acknowledging that you've given yourself
The gift of a few moments of time
To experience the here
And now.

Increasing meditation duration. Try to do at least five minutes of meditation daily, and progress to ten minutes and then fifteen minutes if you can, perhaps over a period of the next two weeks. If doing your meditation without being guided by a tape or CD is too difficult, there are meditation CDs that can be purchased in the stores and our CD, which we use for classes, is now available at www.painspeaking.com. (See recommended reading at the back of the book.)

Walking Meditation When Agitated or Anxious

If you're just too agitated to do a sitting or lying down meditation, you can try a walking meditation instead. Just walk slowly about ten paces, before you slowly and mindfully turn to face the opposite direction and return, and then repeat the process. Or you may walk in a circle if space permits. Keep your eyes open, and keep your attention on your breath or the movement of your legs and feet, aware of being present in each moment.

If you have flashbacks or difficult memories or emotions that come up during a sitting meditation, definitely try the walking meditation. Share your experience with your physician or your therapist, if you have one. Flashbacks or difficult memories don't happen to many, but if you do have this experience, it's important not to shy away from doing the work of meditation: it is likely that those same difficult feelings underlie why you are having such difficulty with pain and healing.

Walking meditation is an active alternative to other types of meditation even when you are too agitated to do a sitting or lying down meditation. These meditations can be very helpful and calming; especially if you have been rushing around and find it hard to settle into a less active position.

Derek's Story

Derek, a tall attractive man in his thirties, was very pleased to see us when he first arrived at the pain clinic. His family physician had assured him we would do a better job at helping him with his pain than his medications were doing. He had suffered a back injury that had kept him out of work for almost seven years and it had not improved, even after four back surgeries. While we were taking his history, he told us there had been a lot of stress in his family.

He had two siblings who were drug addicts and another who was in jail for homicide. He was not an addict, having been put off drugs by witnessing the devastation they had caused in his family. Derek looked as though he carried the weight of the world on his shoulders as he talked about his second marriage and the child he was very proud of, but he was also ashamed of being unable to provide for his family.

We altered his medications to see if we could improve his pain control and tentatively brought up the subject of the mindfulness courses, aware that he might think we were a little crazy for suggesting it to him. To our surprise Derek was interested, although skeptical. He had studied some martial arts in his younger days and believed in mind-body connections. So he went on the list for the next class. We weren't confident that he would attend as he would have a journey of an hour and a half to get to each weekly class.

Derek showed up on the first day of class and sat on the floor, leaning his painful back against the wall. He radiated pain. At the end of the meditation he commented in some surprise that his pain had lessened. Maybe there was something to this, but he still remained skeptical. We didn't expect to see him the following week.

We entered the room the following week to find Derek in his place on the floor leaning against the wall. As requested, he had done a meditation every day working with the CD we had given to him, and he had started to notice a difference. He was calmer and more relaxed at the end of the second class on meditation. He was willing to give this a try. Over the next few classes, he said his wife had noticed that he was more patient. His marriage was improving along with his pain control.

Somewhere around his sixth class, Derek had a meltdown toward the end of the session. His issues with his siblings had really come to the surface. He was too upset to meditate. We doubted that Derek would be back. We phoned him during the seventh week. He was in a quiet state, but disturbed. He didn't know if he would make it to the next class. But he did. We suggested he should try the walking meditation if he was too agitated to do his regular meditation, but in the next couple of weeks, as the weather got warmer, he took his boat out onto the lake and meditated there.

One day he walked into class with resolve: He had got past his difficulty and had decided to change how he dealt with his family members in the future. He didn't have to let them ruin his life. That could happen only if he allowed it!

Classes finished for the summer and in the fall, Derek joined us by attending with other pain sufferers at his local hospital site and linked with us through the magic of telemedicine. He made no secret of the fact that mindfulness had become a hugely important part of his life. He was feeling so much better that he'd chosen to reduce his pain medications. A few weeks later, one of his siblings *was again in trouble with the law. But Derek was dealing with crises better this time around.*

By the time Christmas rolled around, Derek had an announcement. He was off all his pain meds and had started to run; he ran only a short distance but his running was now a few kilometers a day. He emphasized that his having a background in martial arts had helped, because he did not want other people to feel discouraged if they could not do as well.

One year later, Derek was still off medication. Three years later, he is no longer attending our classes, has a job, and has added a second child to his family. He still has pain but it does not rule or ruin his life. He is still meditating daily.

Useful Guidelines for Meditation

The following suggestions will most likely help you as you continue your practice of meditating daily.

Nonstriving. Mindfulness is being fully aware in the present moment as best you can. When your mind wanders, as it inevitably will, you can note whether it causes you to "try" harder. Trying implies opposition and struggle against, which you may not succeed at. So as you note this tendency, you might say to yourself: "It is my intention to stay focused, and every time my mind wanders, I accept the fact that this wandering mind is an inevitable part of the process. I will not call myself names or condemn myself or my experience. Instead I will renew my intention to stay focused on my breath or whatever else I am focusing on."

Goals. We are a goal-orientated society but that orientation doesn't work so well here. Don't set goals for your meditation practice as that gets in the way of accomplishing anything. But if you absolutely cannot prevent yourself from setting goals for your practice, fine. Set them up and then forget about them. Allow your practice to unfold naturally and in its own time and not how you think it "should" be.

Don't start this work when in crisis. Daily meditation recharges your soul and can keep you steady when crises or tragedy arises. We've found, however, that it's often difficult, if not impossible, to teach people how to start meditating while they are in the midst of a personal crisis. It's like trying to teach people to swim while they've fallen into the water and think they're drowning. Better to learn how to swim ahead of time, so if you do fall into the water, you'll know how to handle it. You will find that consistent practice will help you to weather many storms that arrive in your life.

Consider using a guided scenario from a CD or online. Advanced meditators often prefer to meditate in silence. This is because they guide themselves internally the way the voice on a guided meditation CD guides novices externally. Some people gravitate quickly to silent meditations. Others never do. In the end, it doesn't matter whether you meditate to a sound track or in silence—just as long as you do it.

What to do with your thoughts. The moment you're aware that you have drifted, don't push away the thought. Recognize it, note it, explore it if you choose to for a moment (or maybe longer) then return to your focus: this is how you develop insight. If you repel your thoughts as soon as they arise, you are, in fact, practicing a kind of spiritual-emotional avoidance that neutralizes the benefits of mindfulness practice.

Duration of time to meditate. Once you have started a daily practice, there is no single ideal amount of time you "should" be meditating. Some say they feel best doing five-minute meditations at various intervals throughout the day. Others prefer the longer, more structured practice. The important thing to remember is there are no rules, and to do whatever works best for you.

Taking time out from your other commitments. Meditation is a powerful tool. Remember, no matter how much time meditation practice takes out of your day, it usually unclutters your mind and helps you to organize your time so much more effectively, that your productive output increases. One is never too busy to meditate. If busy, meditation helps you to accomplish your daily tasks smoothly, effectively, and with less effort.

next steps

We suggest you spend the next couple of weeks practicing meditation and getting used to seeing the world through more mindful and less judgmental eyes. Make notes in your loose-leaf binder about any difficulties you might encounter. Order CDs if you need them to help you with your formal practice. Take on the challenge and adventure of really becoming intimately aware of the world around you and within you, and of being present for every aspect of your life unfolding.

Chapter 4 will look at your progress with mindfulness, hopefully, after you have been practicing a daily meditation for a couple of weeks.

mindfulness: checking in on your progress

When Mindfulness embraces those we love, they will bloom like flowers.

—Thich Nhat Hahn

We hope you are returning to this chapter after practicing mindfulness for a couple of weeks, as it was described in chapters 2 and 3. Now we intend to check on your progress, offer more guidance, and add further suggestions for you to try.

Did you find you were doing lots of judging when you remembered to look? For example, when you were waiting in the supermarket checkout line ("What's that woman doing? She's being so slow." "He's got ten items to check out and this is the eight items or under line."); or on the road ("What an awful driver!"); and of yourself ("I'm such an idiot, I forgot to take the rental movies back on time again"). And did you note how much your body tenses and tightens when you're annoyed? Start to steam while standing in the checkout line, and your painful back is likely to hurt even worse once you reach the parking lot.

It's quite stressful being judgmental, and you will likely feel much calmer when you're not judging as much. There's a difference between judging whether a meal is good or bad versus flavorful or a little bland, and whether a dress is awful or great versus "right for work" but not for evening wear. Being mindfully aware of this constant tendency to judge, your thoughts of whether something is good or bad (a form of destructive shorthand) may instead become, discerning evaluations or descriptions, which are much less stressful and also very necessary and useful. The judgments as to whether something is good or bad are what cause us to tense, get steamed up, and jar our bodies painfully.

These reactions can be bad for your health and can exacerbate your pain when done continually. Much of our judging is about things that are too insignificant to waste as much energy on as we put into them. When you become aware of what you're doing, it is likely that change will come about without your even needing to try or force the issue.

what makes your pain better? what makes it worse?

Now, let's move to noting what makes your pain increase and what makes it decrease. You may be very comfortable with this homework as it's a typical question asked by doctors. You also may relate to the usual feedback from our patients, which includes increased activity, running low on pain medications, mowing the lawn, arguing with the neighbors, and difficulties with coworkers.

Marla's Story

I didn't realize till I did this homework. I have irritable bowel syndrome. I'd say it got a lot worse about eighteen months ago. I walk a few blocks to work every day. For about the last block or two, my stomach would really start to give me trouble. But last week that didn't happen at all.

Eighteen months ago, one of my colleagues went on maternity leave, and I don't get along with the person who replaced her and now sits at the next desk. I find her moody and condescending. And a new boss arrived a week or two after my colleague was replaced and she really wasn't a good "people person." In fact I'm afraid of her. But last week they were both on vacation. And I noticed that my stomach was feeling much better.

When you really pay attention, you may be surprised at how many social situations exacerbate your pain, rather than just the physical activities you may have easily noticed. For example, Christmas and other holiday situations when families traditionally congregate may cause you great apprehension as you anticipate the difficult emotions that are likely to arise around relatives. They may think you are making too much of your pain and disability. Or they may have well-meaning advice or their presence may bring up old, emotionally painful memories of difficult interactions with them in the past. We're betting your physical pain even ramps up just at the thought of these events. Chapter 9 addresses these issues and will help you to deal with difficult people, especially relatives.

Pacing Your Activities Mindfully

Activity, length of time standing or sitting, and walking are the most frequently noted pain exacerbators. Once you notice that standing for more than twenty minutes at one time increases your back pain, without becoming frustrated, and without allowing a thought like "I feel like a loser" to take root, you simply sit or change your position every twenty minutes. Observing without being judgmental takes the sting out of becoming aware of your need to do this and you will have taken a small step forward. This is also one of the earliest exercises in the "A" word, as some coyly refer to acceptance.

Acceptance. Acceptance that this is the way it is in *this* moment doesn't mean that this is the way it will be forever. Paradoxically, once you arrive at that point of acceptance, research has shown that you may be more likely to improve (McCracken and Eccleston 2005), and acceptance is particularly useful for increasing your physical abilities beyond what you thought you could accomplish. Perhaps it is ironic that the energy spent on your negative emotions when you encounter a task that you could do so easily before your disabling event, and can't do so easily now, can be better spent on healing, strengthening, and adapting. Frustration, anger, and denial are part of the bereavement process for the way you were before your illness, accident or injury. So go ahead, you may need to feel bereaved, but just don't do it for too long.

Take breaks when you need them. Getting an activity or task done by taking breaks when you need to, or by asking for help with parts of it, still gets the task done. And it will be nice not to hurt as much as you did in the past when you *mindlessly* pushed yourself to complete tasks without taking breaks.

Stress-Induced Physical Pain Is Real

It's important to understand that when you hurt, whether it's due to a psychological stress, such as an argument or to increased activity, it really *is* happening physically: there is a physical change at the site where your pain originates. It may be that due to stress hormones circulating throughout your immune system, some inflammation has started up again at the site of your damaged part.

Muscles may be tensing and pushing against neighboring blood vessels, reducing blood flow to the damaged nerves at the site of your pain, causing them to become irritable and to send pain messages to your brain. Perhaps the best example of this process is a migraine headache. After a stressful event, the blood vessels in the head narrow and then expand, and blood flow through them increases and pulses against neighboring structures causing excruciating pain.

So it's not an imaginary pain just because anxious thoughts are at the origin of the discomfort. In fact, wherever your weak spot is located is exactly the place your negative emotions may zero-in to remind you that you're vulnerable. It's as if there's a long telephone wire from your brain to the painful site in your body, with the messages readjusting the activity constantly, depending on how you feel and what you're thinking. The painful part of you increases in intensity like a silent scream from your body: "My system is out of balance again so I hurt!" It's an alert to encourage you to focus on recovery from the latest physical or emotional stressor so that your body systems can function as near normally again, as soon as possible. When the body is malfunctioning, it's likely there is always a reason. Sometimes you can notice and respond; sometimes you can't. If you increase your stress resilience—and mindfulness helps with this—your body is going to recover faster no matter what challenges you are facing.

That Gut Feeling

Sometimes, I (JGN) use a personal anecdote about what happened to me whenever I had exams in medical school to illustrate the mind-body connection. In those instances, my mind used my body—in this case my gut—in a very physical way, to tell me danger was imminent and I should be afraid: very afraid.

I didn't feel that I was in a huge panic before exams. Usually, it was my couch that the high achievers in my year slept on in the week leading up to exams, having their meltdowns, and sure they were going to flunk. Those of us who were less likely to be at the top of the class seemed to be the very people the high achievers came to for comfort and improvised psychotherapy.

Yet, despite being prepared for every exam, from the moment I got up on the morning of the test, but only until the exact moment I put pen to paper, I had diarrhea. And I always worried about what I would do and the time I would lose to reach the bathroom during the exam—but I never needed to reach the bathroom. It was as if the exam anxiety in my mind was displaced directly to my gut: my mind was out of the loop. So my intestine was letting me know that my system was out of balance, but I couldn't do anything about it. The exams had to be done.

---

continuing to practice mindfulness

Being present for day-to-day activities really does help your physical pain because when you are fully present for that activity, you're not so focused on your pain, and with continuing mindfulness practice, you become even safer and less clumsy. The following sections present ideas on how you can continue to practice mindfulness.

Showering Mindfully

Have you ever taken the time to notice what a luxury to your senses the shower provides? Often you're in the shower with the entire office staff or your family (in your mind), and you don't really notice anything about the experience itself. Taking a shower can provide an opportunity to tune in to your senses and enjoy the feeling of the warm spray of water, the fragrance of the soap, and the feel of the shampoo as you lather your hair. Being fully present with the temperature of the water, the feeling of the towels, the experience of having time to yourself: all of this is a mindfulness experience not to be missed.

Cleaning Mindfully

Whether it is the simple act of dusting, vacuuming, doing the wash, or cleaning out the cat box, you can revisit your old tasks and see them as opportunities to be mindful.

Cleaning out your fridge—a task you might hate—becomes transformed when you focus your energies. In the past, perhaps you put off the task thinking that you had other more important things to do. But, in fact, all you have is now. All you ever have is now. Life is one long continuous now and there is no now that brings with it a greater sense of importance or meaning than another now: all nows are important.

As you wash dishes, you can turn your attention to the scent of the liquid soap, the feeling of the cloth in your hand, and the feeling of the surface of the plate as it is cleansed. You can enjoy the feeling of orderliness and accomplishment. The dishwashing may bring you back to what is important, to be here, in the now, fully present, without judging one moment as more important than another moment.

Cleaning out your spices can become a celebration for your senses. You can explore the scent of each spice, enjoy its fragrance, or decide whether it is too old to be of any further use in your kitchen, and discard or retain it as you gauge each spice's potency.

Clearing clutter can be an overwhelming task. Clutter can fill your home distracting you from the present. The piles of clothes that no longer fit, the bits of broken china, or old objects you no longer use or need—all are tied in with your past and may be becoming symbols of past accomplishments or regrets. Clearing clutter mindfully can be done in short manageable time periods: even fifteen minutes at a time, over many months. It can bring you back in line with what's important now, what's right for now as you choose to let go of what is no longer important. Doing this activity mindfully helps you respond more fully to the present and allows you to fill your living space with only those items that you need and want now.

distraction—or less pain?

When you become more mindful, your pain often feels as though it has decreased. The question is: does the pain diminish because you are being distracted from it, so you're not noticing it, or does the pain really decrease? Actually, the definition of *pain* is that it is an unpleasant sensation that the mind notices. So, if your mind is noticing less pain, your pain *has* decreased. You are not just being distracted from it. If your mind is engaged elsewhere, the activity in your brain areas that register pain is reduced, so the pain is truly lessened. This has been supported by functional MRI studies such as those done by Catherine Bushnell and her colleagues at McGill University in Montreal (Villemure et al. 2003).

As you become more used to paying attention to what you're experiencing, you will find that stringing mindful activities together is like threading beads onto a string. Eventually, you see a beautiful necklace and you can't see the string. Similarly, with one mindful activity following the next, your moments of noticing pain lessen as you truly pay attention to your moments, engaged in other experiences. In chapter 5, we'll have a look at your progress, so far, with the formal practice of mindfulness.

Chapter 5

meditation challenges

Challenge is a dragon with a gift in its mouth.
Tame the dragon and the gift is yours.

—Noela Evans

By now, you've had the opportunity to start to practice formal meditation for some time and you may have encountered various difficulties along the way. This chapter will review some of the more common challenges that can arise.

increased mental restlessness: or monkey mind

One common complaint from those who are just beginning to practice meditation is that the very attempt to concentrate results in a greater restlessness of mind. Sometimes this happens because it is only when you start to meditate that you realize how active your mind is. You become aware of all the thoughts and feelings that are normally there, but you've never paid attention to them before, and you may think that your mind is getting noisier or more agitated than it ever was previously. However, this may be an indication that your mind is becoming quieter. You're just becoming aware of how noisy and demanding your thoughts and feelings have always been. Most likely your mind was all over the place most of the time. Meditation allows you to see and reduce the amount of chatter your mind engages in. It induces a state of relaxed alertness that can also be called *thought awareness*.

As thoughts arise that have nothing to do with your breath (and this is inevitable), you don't have to get angry or impatient with yourself. Acknowledge that you have lost focus and without making judgments about yourself, gently return the focus of your attention to your breath. Witnessing what distracts you will give you insight and actually takes you a step closer to maintaining your focus. So, when you experience the chattering of what is called the *monkey mind*, the best way to handle this situation is simply to examine the thoughts, then let them go, and return your mind to the focus you are attending to.

Timing

In the last week did you meditate consistently? Or was it hard to make time in your schedule or find a time when other people would leave you alone? Perhaps you found it difficult to get into a consistent routine. Consider talking to family members to get them to cooperate so you can take some uninterrupted time out to do your formal meditation. Sometimes family members see the benefits of daily meditation in you before you do. If that happens, a family member may remind you, "Isn't it time for you to do your meditation today?"

A consistent time every day works for some people, especially if you find yourself going to bed at night having not "got around to doing it." If you have a tendency to fall asleep during meditation, which is a fairly common initial observation, perhaps meditating first thing in the morning might work better for you.

If you are in the workforce, meditating straight after work on arriving home might work better for you. If you are pressed for time at the beginning or end of the workday, you can try using your car at lunchtime. Park it somewhere quiet, and meditate. But we must emphasize this: please don't meditate while driving. Don't even think about doing that!

Kids and Pets

Young children and pets are sometimes a problem for meditators, but some people find that their pets eventually get into the habit of lying down quietly when their owner is meditating and doing it too. Or they leave their pets outside the bedroom door while meditation is in progress. Older kids sometimes join a parent for the meditation.

Meditating early in the morning before the younger kids wake up, or when they're at school, or when you're waiting for them in the car outside their extracurricular activities are all options you could try. We remember the delightful picture presented by Saki Santorelli, who took over running the Mindfulness Program at Massachusetts Medical School from Jon Kabat-Zinn. Saki would meditate every morning sitting cross-legged on the floor with a big blanket wrapped around him, into which one of his small children would occasionally disappear, as if it were a wigwam.

Falling Asleep

Falling asleep is another common concern. If this is an issue for you, perhaps you could try meditating in a sitting position rather than lying down, or during the day rather than in the evening. If you are already sleep-deprived and meditation is helping you to sleep, we say "go for it" because sleep deprivation makes pain worse and it's harder to cope. But then it is advisable to add a meditation earlier in the day, and see if you can stay awake and alert for that.

If you can never stay awake meditating even while sitting, you still can do all your formal practice as walking meditation, or as yoga postures, or as mindful movements, which are described in chapter 7. Falling asleep during meditation might be a defense mechanism against pain, or a sign of the intense sleep deprivation that many of our chronic pain patients suffer due to their pain or to the side effects of their medications.

Noisy Environments

At first, you might find that noise disturbs you, but as you become more practiced at meditating you may find that you can meditate through noise, and even make it part of your meditation experience. However, this is not so likely when you are new to meditation. Pneumatic drills outside in the street will understandably cause difficulty, but with practice even that might become possible for you.

The Hospital Fire Alarm

One day when we were in the third week of class, we were meditating as the fire alarm started its piercing shriek through the hospital's loudspeaker system. As usual, I made note of the fact that in a healing institution it seems insane to me to have such a disruptive noise—a different tone surely could be just as useful in its capacity to alert—and I had a mental picture of every hospital patient's immune system halting in its tracks due to the stress of the noise.

But as it started, I noted that class participants to my right had not moved a muscle and those to my left had jumped. The difference was those to my right were alumni and had been practicing meditation for several months and those to my left were "newbies."

Avoid Meditating When You Have Too Much Pain or Too Much Medication

Finding the right time to practice formal meditation also involves choosing a time when your pain is not at its worst. Remember, you're not doing it to get out of pain. Your pain may recede when you meditate, but it also may not. You may know that a couple of hours after a dose of medication you are in your best pain-controlled time: that may be the best time to settle down for a meditation. But if medication makes you drowsy or gives you brain fog, it is going to work against the clear mind you can achieve with meditation, and you may not get as much out of it. For example, high doses of some of the anticonvulsants taken for pain can keep you from getting the most out of the meditative work.

Sometimes patients in our practice have reported their minds are more cloudy than normal because of their medications, and they especially notice the difference if they are able to come off of pain medications after doing this work. They report getting more out of the meditation and mindfulness when they have a clearer mind. In those circumstances, and if you feel you are making progress and might manage with less medication, it's certainly worth discussing with your prescribing physician whether cutting down on your medication very slowly would be advisable, so that you can get the most out of this work with your mind.

Emotional Stress

The purpose of meditation is to "show up" in your own life, and not necessarily to feel good. We live in a culture that has a phobia about suffering. Advertisements everywhere tell us how to be happy. By and large, suffering is seen as something we must try to escape. We're not particular fans of suffering ourselves but we do know that by paying attention to our suffering we can learn many beneficial lessons. If during meditation practice, you find the suffering too great to bear, note it, and move on. Return to it again later, when you feel stronger. But don't avoid it altogether; suffering has much to teach us.

At times of major stress in your life, you may not feel very motivated to practice meditation and mindfulness, but those times are also times that not much can be done to help manage your pain with medication. Medication is not likely to work as well when your stress is intense, and your sleep is of poor quality. So, at times of increased stress it may feel as though it may not be possible to meditate at all, especially if you are new to it; however, there is an alternative: movement meditation like walking meditation, yoga, or mindful movements (see chapter 7) might work the best for you.

Battling with insurers, employers, and courts can be a terrible time overloaded with stress. However, once settlements have been reached and you know what your financial outlook is likely to be, progress can be made. Both mindfulness and pain often become more manageable, and you may even be able to move forward and improve.

It's such a catch-22 situation! When lawyers ask us if a patient is likely to get any better than he or she is right now, and will the patient ever be able to join the workforce again, the lawyers don't really want to hear, "Well, once the stress of this case is over, and this patient knows what his or her financial situation will be in the future, the patient will likely improve; and whether he or she can ever work again is more likely to have a positive answer once this nightmare has ended!"

Getting better after legal or insurance battles are over is not malingering. It's very difficult to have a positive attitude about your future and your ability to rehabilitate when you are fighting a large organization for money to put food on the table and a roof over your head.

flashbacks and anxiety

We truly believe that frequently there are past events, often as far back as childhood, that underlie the inability of the body to heal in a timely fashion. If you've had a trauma that had a huge impact in your past, during meditation those memories may rise to the surface. After all, now that there are fewer distractions, your mind is clearer. If such memories come to you, they likely need to be observed. However, you can start by mindfully "sitting" with acknowledging they are there; at first, perhaps under the surface of your mind. Allow them to come into focus gradually over several sittings. There's no need to struggle with what to do with painful memories. Just sit with them.

If such thoughts and memories are too troubling, discuss them with your physician or therapist. As they bubble to the surface of your mind, they may need some work, which you might or might not be able to do alone. But resist the urge to stuff them back down into your subconscious mind. This is such an opportunity to move forward, beyond them, because, assuredly, they weren't doing you any good when they were stuck in your subconscious. Such memories are like an infection deep within a surgical wound: we can suture over the top, but a wound never heals properly until the infection is cleared out from the bottom up; only then will it heal.

By witnessing many people in our classes going through this process, we've come to realize that sometimes people are more scared of feeling emotional pain than they are of physical pain. In fact, sometimes the physical pain is a distraction from feeling the emotional pain and is easier to bear; and, unfortunately, physical pain is a more "legitimate" pain to the outside world. After all, it's more acceptable to tell your employer that you have a migraine and need to go home than to say you feel too depressed to work and need to leave. And, sometimes, it seems as if your body knows this and helps you along by translating your emotional distress into the physical pain, for example, of a migraine.

committing to daily meditation

If you live alone, have few commitments, and have not established a routine for meditating, do you still find that by bedtime you haven't yet found the time to meditate? It's sad to say, but true, that the less we have to do, the less we do. This is another form of deconditioning in addition to the weakening of the muscles that you aren't using. If this is so for you, we ask that you observe it as a fact. Don't jump on the mind train to despondency and depression about it. All you need to do is find a consistent time of day to sit formally and commit to a specific time period to meditate.

introducing a nonstriving attitude

Most importantly, after making the commitment, it is then best just to sit with whatever comes up during your meditation and not strive to get anywhere with it. Solutions and progress find you during your practice; not the other way round. For example, you may have noticed that sometimes when you wake in the morning, a solution came to you while you slept. The same process is true for meditation. Meditation and sleep share some similarities in what they can do for your mind and body.

Meditation: The Reset Button

We believe that meditation, like sleep, provides a reset button for stress that was accumulated throughout the previous day. It you have been idle because of your chronic pain, note that being underutilized can be as stressful as being too busy. Mindfully, this practice may help you to take baby steps toward taking up new activities, reducing your fear that you might fail at them even before you start. And meditation is portable: you can take it with you wherever you go. To paraphrase the title of one of Jon Kabat-Zinn's books: wherever you go, there it is! You can meditate in a waiting room, on an aircraft, in an MRI scanner, and even in a dental chair.

In the next chapter we'll revisit the brain again; the seat of your mind. And we will turn on the flashlight for another look around to help you understand what you are doing as you continue to work with your inner resources.

Chapter 6

searching the brain for clues to pain: turning on that flashlight

The human brain is the most complex object in the universe. It works closely with the second most complex object in the universe—the human body.

—John J. Ratey, MD

In this chapter we'll take a deeper look at what is going on in your mind and body when you continually feel pain. The belief that your mind plays an important role in physical illness goes back to the earliest days of medicine. From the time of the ancient Greeks, it was generally accepted that the person's state of mind affected the course of an illness and was an important consideration in the treatment of disease. Candace Pert in her book *Molecules of Emotion* (1997), recounted that this understanding changed in the seventeenth-century when the philosopher and founding father of modern medicine, René Descartes, wanted to obtain human bodies for dissection. At that time, the Catholic Church forbade human dissection, believing it would violate the soul, which was believed to reside in and throughout the body.

Descartes, however, proposed a novel theory. He thought that body and soul were two distinctly separate entities entirely unrelated to each other, and that the soul existed exclusively in the head. The Pope agreed, and Descartes was granted permission to dissect cadavers from the neck on down.

It is likely that this long-forgotten "understanding" still influences the thinking of many of today's physicians who believe the mind is separate from the body, and that your mental state has no bearing on your physical wellness. However, the tide has begun to turn as researchers continue to discover the many ways that our brain's response to stress can profoundly influence our body's susceptibility to illness and chronic pain.

what exactly is pain?

Your body is like a finely tuned instrument and the processes involved in sensing pain are extremely complex. For example, if you burn your thumb by touching a hot plate, the chemicals released from the injured cells in your skin travel through fluids over to nerve fibers close to the injury. These nerve fibers have special sites on their surfaces called *receptors* that when contacted by the inflammatory chemicals, trigger an extremely rapid set of reactions. It's sort of like the telephone ringing to alert you to take the call. The chemical changes at the site of your injury cause increases in electrical activity through neighboring small nerve fibers (called *C fibers* and *A-delta fibers*) to take the message to your spine, which then relays the sensation, which is pain, up to your brain.

The area in your brain that is the first to receive all sensory information including pain, touch, sight, and smell is called the *thalamus*; it is just above the base of your brain which sits on top of your spinal column. When the brain of a less evolved animal receives a pain message, it triggers a simple protective reflex for the animal to remove itself from the source of the pain. The thalamus sends an instant message to the motor center in the less evolved back brain (where automatic functions, such as breathing and heart rate, are governed), ensuring the animal will try to protect itself from further pain by moving away from the source of the pain, if it can. The brain also immediately starts to manufacture internal painkillers called *endorphins*, which act like morphine or opioids. This is partly why after the most intense pain is felt, the pain often dies down quickly. When the threat is intense, this fast reaction is essential for survival.

the human brain

In humans, however, the pain responses are more complex than they are in less evolved animals. If you can, hold up your right hand in front of you, cross your thumb across your palm and make a fist over it, bending the fist slightly forward at the wrist. Now, imagine your arm is your spinal cord. Your thumb represents the less evolved hind brain, which is responsible for basic life functions such as breathing and maintaining your heartbeat—the more automatic functioning of your organs—and reflex reactions like removing your hand from an intense heat source.

The fist represents the next stage of evolution: the *limbic system*, which evolved into the emotional centers and senses. The limbic system originally started with the development of the smell-sensing olfactory lobe, which was very important for safety, and is very highly developed in many animals. The thalamus, which registers sight, touch, and pain as well as other functions, is a part of the limbic system.

The *amygdala* and *hippocampus* are two other parts of the brain within the limbic system. During evolution, the hippocampus became involved in the ability to learn and to memorize, and the amygdala became the part of the brain that registered emotions. Today, when something triggers an emotional reaction, the hippocampus remembers the context, and the amygdala registers the uncensored emotion.

So when a small child looks at a hot plate, her hippocampus remembers that the last time she touched the hot plate she burned her thumb, and that the hot plate is therefore dangerous. At the same time, her amygdala might send a surge of fear through her body as a memory of what happened the last time she touched the hot plate.

There are direct connections between the thalamus and the motor centers of our hind brain. These connections create a shortcut between receiving a sensation and physically responding to that sensation to protect ourselves from injury—without any conscious thought being involved. So the small child's thumb is withdrawn quickly from the hot plate, even before the higher centers of her brain have interpreted what is happening.

The Higher Centers of the Human Brain: The Neocortex

Now cup your other hand over your fist. This other hand represents the higher centers of the brain, the *neocortex*, which is the most recently evolved part of the mammalian brain, and governs thought, reasoning, and other executive functions. There are also connections between the thalamus and these higher brain centers. This is where the interpretation of many inputs, including pain, takes place. And our interpretations of these inputs govern our responses, even whether we choose to pay attention or not to the inputs. So these interpretations are decided at a more conscious level and can be modified accordingly.

The neocortex in human beings isn't fully developed until well into our twenties. In an infant or small child, reactions to unpleasant experiences are processed by the amygdala, hippocampus, and other parts of the emotional limbic system with less input from the evolutionarily "newer" or "higher" thought and reasoning centers. We need the neocortex to modify our responses to the emotions that the amygdala processes or else we would not be able to be functioning members of society.

So if you are born into a household where a parent has frequent loud temper tantrums, as a child you might develop a hair-trigger flinching response to any loud noise similar to the noise made by the parent who had temper tantrums. This flinching response can continue on well into your adult life, and you might not even make the connection. Moreover, that response can become a chronic stress reaction with profound implications for your body's resilience to illness—and its ability to repair after an injury later on in your life.

Dr. Jackie's Cat's Flight Reflex

One of my cats was born on a building site where he spent the first eight weeks of his life fending for himself. Many evenings, I sat patiently on the step at my backdoor during the early weeks of his life to get him to begin trusting me when he came looking for food, which he did regularly. Eventually, if I moved very slowly, he overcame his hair-trigger reaction to flee every time I came within touching distance. Eventually, I managed to catch him to take him to the vet to get his shots, deworming, etc., so I could bring him inside to join our family as a pet. But nine years later, he has never lost his reflex to flee from any unusual circumstance, and even from some not so unusual events. For example, he disappears under couches whenever anyone unknown to him enters our home, and he will stay there for hours. His instant flight reflexes were imprinted during those first eight weeks of his life. When we moved into another house, he disappeared and hid in the basement for three days!

We believe there is a similar reflex in humans who have endured adverse events in their very early lives; it is a reflex that affects all body functions when accidents or injuries or other challenges to the body occur later in life.

your body's protection systems

Your body is endowed with protection systems for the maintenance of life. One of these is the system that mobilizes protection against threats to your well-being. It is called the *hypothalamus-pituitary-adrenal (HPA) axis*. When there are no threats, the HPA axis is "quiet," and your growth and the maintenance of your various systems continue functioning as usual. However, when the hypothalamus in your brain perceives an external or an internal threat, the HPA axis unleashes a cascade of chemical responses that trigger the fight-or-flight response, often resulting in a heightened susceptibility to illness and a decreased ability to heal from that illness. How does that happen?

The Hypothalamus-Pituitary-Adrenal (HPA) Axis: The Fight-or-Flight Response

Stresses that trigger the HPA axis cause a simple domino effect. This is how it works: Your hypothalamus secretes a chemical called *corticotrophin-releasing factor* (CRF) that travels to your pituitary gland causing it to release *adrenocorticotropic hormone* (ACTH) into the blood. ACTH then makes its way to your *adrenal* glands, which sit on top of your kidneys, where it turns on the secretion of your fight-or-flight adrenal hormones: *cortisol* and *adrenaline*. These two stress hormones coordinate the functioning of your body's organs, providing you with great physiological power to fend off or flee danger.

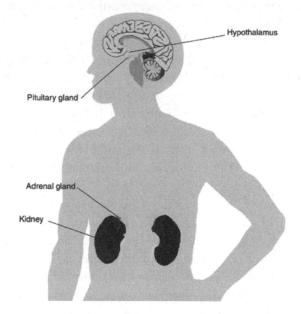

Figure 6.1: *The hypothalamus-pituitary-adrenal (HPA) axis*

These stress hormones circulate in your blood, speed up your heart rate, increase your breathing rate, constrict the blood vessels of your digestive tract, and divert energy-providing blood from your digestive tract to the muscles of your arms and legs to enable you to get out of harm's way fast. Your digestive organs stop doing their life-sustaining work of digestion, absorption, excretion, and other functions that provide for the growth of your cells and the production of your body's energy reserves. This is okay for a short amount of time, allowing you to "outrun the tiger," but if the perception of threat becomes chronic, this same stress response inhibits the growth of cells and other maintenance processes and further compromises your body's survival and well-being. It's easy to see why we get nauseated when stressed, and how irritable bowel syndrome starts.

The HPA Axis and Its Effects on the Immune System

Your stress hormones such as cortisol affect another protection system in your body, the immune system. The immune system protects the body from internal threats, such as infections caused by bacteria and viruses and early cancer cells, in addition to doing tissue-damage repair. To get a sense of how much energy the immune system uses, recall how weak you become when you are fighting infections like a cold or flu.

Why does the adrenal system shut down your immune system? Well, imagine you are being hunted by a tiger. Your unconscious brain processes must decide which is a greater threat: the immediate danger of the tiger who is about to leap and devour you, or the longer-term threat of infection or tissue damage. Clearly, the immediate threat is a greater danger. But you can see why engaging the HPA axis chronically has the secondary consequence of interfering with our ability to fight disease and repair our tissues.

Dr. Janice Kiecolt-Glaser and her husband Dr. Ronald Glaser reported in 2003 that small wounds took an average of nine days longer to heal in women who cared for patients with Alzheimer's disease than in women who were not under similar stress. In another study, which they reported in 2004, arguments between husbands and wives were accompanied by increases in stress hormones and immunological changes over a twenty-four-hour period (Heffner et al. 2004). Stress also seems to make people more likely to contract some infectious illnesses. Dr. Sheldon Cohen and his colleagues at Carnegie Mellon have spent years inoculating intrepid volunteers with cold and influenza viruses, and their findings, reported in 2006, offer strong evidence that stressed people are more likely to become infected and to have more severe symptoms after becoming ill.

The HPA Axis and Its Effect on the Neocortex

Activating the HPA axis also interferes with your ability to think clearly and sleep soundly. Sound sleep is essential for the immune system to function and repair the body properly, for clear thinking, and even for maintaining balance. In an emergency, the additional blood flow serves to activate your hind brain, which is the source of the life-sustaining reflexes that most effectively control your fight-or-flight behavior (Takamatsu et al. 2003; Arnsten and Goldman-Rakic 1998; Goldstein et al. 1996).

the heavy cost of chronic stress

In 2002, Dr. Bruce S. McEwen, director of the neuroendocrinology laboratory at Rockefeller University and author of *The End of Stress as We Know It* reported that prolonged or severe stress can weaken your immune system, strain your heart, damage memory cells in your brain, and deposit fat at your waist rather than your hips and buttocks, which is a risk factor for heart disease, cancer, and other illnesses. Stress has also been implicated in irritable bowel disease, aging, depression, heart disease, rheumatoid arthritis, diabetes, and many other illnesses and painful conditions.

Dr. McEwen points out that your capacity to manage stress is influenced by your heredity and childhood experiences; by your diet, exercise, and sleep patterns; by the presence or absence of close personal relationships; by your income level and social status, and by encountering a number of simultaneous stresses to the point that they overload your system. In moderate amounts stress can be benign, even beneficial, and most people are equipped to deal with it. It is harmful only when it overloads your system.

He conducted research in rats to demonstrate this wear-and-tear effect. The rats were subjected to increased levels of stress by handling them during their normal resting time and placing them in a small compartment that restricted their movement for six hours a day. On the first day that the rats were restrained, their cortisol levels rose in line with their stress response. In later days, however, their cortisol production would switch off earlier each day as they became more accustomed to being handled. At twenty-one days, the rats began to grow anxious and became aggressive, common effects of chronic stress. Their immune systems became slower to fight off invaders, the nerve cells in their hippocampuses (the brain region involved in memory) atrophied, and they stopped producing new hippocampal neurons (McEwen, Liston, and Morrison 2006).

Dr. McEwen points out that stress is often worsened by how you respond to stress. For example, you might eat fatty foods, stay late at work, avoid exercise, sleep less, and smoke or drink more. And because high levels of cortisol can actually shrink nerve cells in the hippocampus, there can also be some changes in memory that are more typically associated with aging. Some evidence also links a smaller hippocampus with post-traumatic stress disorder, depression, and sexual abuse in childhood, although the meaning of this size difference is still being debated.

Like all other hormones in the human body, cortisol normally rises and falls with daily rhythms. Its production is higher in the morning and lower in the evening. Prolonged or severe stress appears to disrupt this cycle giving you a higher baseline cortisol level, as well as producing too much or too little of it at the wrong times. This would have an impact on your immune system's functioning, your ability to repair damaged parts of your body, and therefore, your likelihood of suffering pain.

The Risk from Early Exposure to Stress: Lifelong Effects

Why do some people seem more vulnerable to life's pressures than others? Among other reasons, personality and health habits play a role. Moreover, severe stress in early life appears to cast a long shadow. Dr. Michael Meaney of McGill University and his colleagues found that rat pups that were intensively groomed and licked by their mothers as infants were bolder and secreted lower levels of the stress hormone ACTH in stressful situations than rats that had lacked such attention—a benefit that lasted throughout their lives (Meaney and Szyf 2005).

In humans, physical and sexual abuse and other traumas in childhood have been associated with a more pronounced response to stress later in life. In a study done by Dr. Charles Nemeroff, a psychiatrist at Emory University, and his colleagues (Heim et al. 2000), they found that women who had been physically or sexually abused as children secreted more of the two stress hormones in response to a mildly stressful situation than women who had not been abused.

Perhaps the best indicator of how people are likely to be affected by stress is their position in the social hierarchy. In subordinate male monkeys, for example, the stress of constantly being servile to their alpha, dominant counterparts causes damage in the hippocampus. And dominant monkeys who are repeatedly moved from social group to social group, thus forcing them to constantly reestablish their dominance, also exhibit severe stress and are more likely to develop *atherosclerosis* (hardening of the arteries), according to studies by Dr. Jay Kaplan of Wake Forest University School of Medicine and colleagues (Miller-Butterworth et al. 2008). It would be pleasing to think that humans are less chained to their social rankings than monkeys, but studies repeatedly show that the risk for many diseases increases with every step down the socioeconomic scale, even when factors like smoking, diet, and access to health care have been taken into account (McEwen and Lasley 2002).

Short-Term Stress Triggers Natural Pain Relievers

In the short term, stress can be a powerful painkiller. When your brain senses a serious threat or a traumatic injury, it releases a veritable pharmacy of chemicals to quickly dampen the pain. Called *stress-induced analgesia*, this reaction explains why often you don't feel pain immediately following an injury. Stress-induced analgesia enables a soldier in the midst of a battle to focus on survival rather than pain, and a person who has suffered a broken leg in an accident is enabled to walk on that leg, if necessary, immediately after the bone has been broken.

Interestingly, the painkillers released by your body during stressful situations are very similar to the chemicals found in illicit drugs. In addition to blocking pain, these chemicals trigger the release of *dopamine*, a neurotransmitter that provides feelings of pleasure. In 2005, researcher Andrea Hohmann and her associates discovered that stress can also trigger the release of marijuana-like compounds called *cannabinoids*. The study, published in *Nature*, found that the body's version of marijuana is also effective at blocking pain.

When used *long term* for continuing pain, opioids (narcotics) are now thought to block the natural painkilling mechanisms in *some* individuals, a phenomenon, called *hyperalgesia*. So they may begin to feel more pain than other people who are not on painkillers, and tapering off their drugs may actually improve their pain management.

Lingering Stress Sets You Up for Chronic Pain

Although your body is well-equipped to block out pain during short periods of stress, its response to long-lasting stress isn't nearly as helpful. The brain cannot keep pumping out internal opioids (*endorphins*) forever, and the supply eventually runs out. To make things worse, stress also damages the brain's ability to produce dopamine, the pleasure compound, which is stimulated by opioids. In short, chronic stress can short-circuit your brain's normal response to adversity.

For some people, this chemical upheaval can set the stage for chronic pain. According to a 2004 report in *Medical Hypotheses* by Patrick Wood, stress-induced damage to the body's dopamine-producing mechanisms may contribute to the onset of *fibromyalgia*. People with this condition are extremely sensitive to pain and often have unexplained pain in trigger points throughout their body. Fibromyalgia may be an exception to a basic rule of stress-related diseases. That is, heart disease, hypertension, depression, and other diseases can get started when the body produces an overload of stress hormones. Fibromyalgia may be just the opposite: as reported by Dr. John McBeth and colleagues in 2005, some studies have found that people with fibromyalgia tend to have unusually low levels of cortisol, the hormone that the body releases in times of stress. The lack of cortisol may be a sign that body isn't responding to stress—or fighting pain—the way it should.

Stress Can Be "Banked"

Healing is not only affected by stress in the here and now, but also by the stress you "banked" in the past and never really dealt with. Because we work with so many chronic pain sufferers who reported severe childhood stressors (for example, parental deaths before they were out of their teens, parental neglect, abuse, substance abuse, and mental illness), we realized that when their essential brain pathways were being formed, there was likely to be something different about their "stress-handling" brain pathways. So if you were subjected to so much stress in childhood and you were also a highly sensitive individual, the odds are even greater that your stress-handling pathways will be abnormal. The young body often appears to cope and remain physically alright despite abnormal stress-handling pathways in the brain; the middle-aged body doesn't.

A landmark study was done in the early 1990s by an American group, Schofferman and his colleagues, who looked at the outcomes of individuals who'd had spinal surgeries (Schofferman et al. 1993). They were asked about their memories of their experiences with their caregivers or parents in the past. Had there been any physical, emotional, or sexual abuse; or had a parent or caregiver been an abuser of alcohol or drugs; or had a parent or caregiver disappeared, either by leaving the household or by dying? For those patients who'd had none of these things happen to them, 95 percent did well after surgery and did not require as much pain relief. For those who remembered three or more of these "risk factors," only 15 percent did well after surgery.

Some individuals manage to escape unscathed from such troubled backgrounds, but many don't. And the casualties are likely to be those with a myriad of health-related problems who are patients at a variety of clinics, including all the specialty clinics in hospital mental health services and addiction services, not just the pain clinics.

Pregnancy and Stress

A frightening number of studies cited in a review by Welberg and Seckl (2001) stated that if your mother had been stressed during her pregnancy with you, then you had been bathed in amniotic fluid containing high levels of the stress hormone cortisol. When a pregnant woman is highly stressed, that can lead to premature birth, lower birth weight, lower IQ of the child, behavioral difficulties, schizophrenia, learning disabilities, autism, diabetes, impaired glucose tolerance, hypertension, and probably many other disorders that haven't been studied yet. A certain amount of stress in pregnancy is important to "prime" the infant, and it's important during our lives too, so we will know how to handle stress, just as it's important for our bodies to be exposed, over time, to manageable or slight infections so that we can build immunity.

Welberg and Seckl's review covers at least three decades of laboratory animal, particularly rat, experiments looking at the effects of maternal stress on the fetus and its long-term effects after birth. They report the effects vary between different strains of rats, but the evidence is compelling, and some correlations have already been seen in human studies. Essentially, their report states that the fetus bathed in high levels of stress hormone in the amniotic fluid is more likely to have a more rapid and sustained stress-hormone response to challenges after birth and throughout life. Females are affected more than males, and the adverse effects of accumulating stress responses during the animals' life spans are more pronounced on health as the animal ages. Stress, remember, affects our ability to heal and repair. When that's impaired we're more likely to suffer chronic pain.

Your body is striving for balance: too much infection and every cell is infected. Well, similarly, too much stress and every cell is affected.

fibromyalgia, stress, and sleep

Fibromyalgia, a disease of pain in many parts of the body, affects women more than men, and in our opinion, is a prime example of the stress response having been abnormally programmed into the developing brain with devastating consequences when the sufferers are in their thirties or forties. In our practice, many people with fibromyalgia report difficult life experiences that affected them in profound ways. Sometimes, they didn't even realize the impact of these early difficult life experiences until they started meditating and learning how to trust in and inhabit awareness itself.

Sleep studies in fibromyalgic individuals usually show they habitually experience a low amount of or even no restorative sleep. Also, they often exhibit brain wave forms called *alpha intrusions*, which means the brain often appears to wake up while asleep several times an hour, without the individual knowing it. Their rapid body responses to stress, deeply etched into the neural paths of their minds and bodies, have become so automatic that these responses are their "normal." They're exhausted because of the lack of restful sleep. And their body repair is suspended or reduced by a poor immune system affected by their chronic stress and lack of sleep, causing sore muscles and joints.

Chronic stress also causes irritability of their bowels (irritable bowel syndrome [IBS]). Their lack of good quality sleep causes brain fog. Your brain becomes pretty foggy if you haven't had any decent sleep for even a couple of nights, and the person with fibromyalgia has likely been experiencing poor sleep for years. Sometimes an accident, injury or surgery precipitates the development of this disease, but the background stressors were already lurking there and waiting for the next stressor to arrive and just take things "over the top."

Fibromyalgia and Gestational Stress

If childhood stress is reported by our patients, it's likely that family stress preceded their birth. Sure enough, Professor Hellhammer, of the University of Trier in Germany, reported to the Sixth International Congress of Neuroendocrinology in 2006 how vulnerable the fetus is to prenatal stress. In a study that looked at ninety-three women with fibromyalgia and compared them with 100 normal female controls, significantly more of the fibromyalgia sufferers reported that their mothers had experienced profound stress during pregnancy. It was reported that, similar to animal studies, their adrenal gland development had likely been impaired, and their stress response was abnormal. Being unable to produce enough cortisol isn't good for the body in ways that are similar to being unable to produce enough insulin is for diabetics. Adequate cortisol production is needed to support all your physiological systems in times of stress.

So, although initially it looked as though fibromyalgia sufferers were suffering from chronically high cortisol levels due to early exposure to chronic stressors, it now looks as though their body systems are under siege from a *deficiency* of stress hormones just when they are most needed. This doesn't lead those with fibromyalgia to becoming laid-back nonstressed people however. It leads to a chronic inability to handle stress, in the same way that untreated diabetics have a high blood sugar content that damages their organs.

persisting pain

When pain messages are sent over and over again from the body part that is damaged, a memory of that pain accumulates in the brain, nerves become hypersensitive; and what might not have been perceived as painful—a light touch, for example—becomes painful. That's why if you have a severe migraine headache, the skin over your skull may be tender to touch; and why a person suffering from the painful condition of fibromyalgia usually finds not very painful challenges much more painful than people without fibromyalgia do.

When you respond to stressors frequently and intensely, remember that your immune system, gut, and the restorative phases of your sleep decrease their activities in the presence of stress hormones, so it's harder to recover from injuries or illness, especially as you age. Not healing from an injury or painful illness is stressful. Being disabled and unable to work is stressful. Worry interferes with sleep which also interferes with recovery. Even some pain and sleep drugs interfere with restorative sleep. Pain interferes with movement and, with restricted movement, muscles get weak; the damaged part of the body has less support from the surrounding muscles and so becomes more painful. Not getting out of the house, not bringing in the same income, not being able to be active, all contribute to becoming depressed. Everything then becomes overwhelming and pain suffering increases.

This is also true of emotional pain: the more stressed you are, the more you react to the next stressor, and the longer you feel it. And so the cycle downward continues.

Proving Pain

"Psychosomatic" has been almost an insulting term used by health professionals to describe a physical condition, such as pain, that they believe has been entirely brought about by psychological causes. But every illness or response to injury has both a physical and psychological component. And when we feel stressed, it can bring on physical illnesses, such as shingles and stomach ulcers.

What really took this understanding forward was the exciting work in the functional magnetic resonance imaging field, some of which was done in Canada, particularly at McGill University in Montreal and Toronto Western Hospital in Toronto. *Functional MRIs* (fMRIs) are a research tool, a way of imaging the brain to show it functioning when engaged in certain activities or states of mind, such as feeling pain. Using these brain scans, similar areas of the brain have been shown to "light up" when either emotional or physical pain is being experienced.

Recent work (Villemure, Slotnick, and Bushnell 2003) has shown that the areas of the brain that light up in response to a painful stimulus can be dulled by creating positive moods with a pleasant odor; the basis of aromatherapy. Unpleasant odors can actually exacerbate physical pain and pain-related areas in the brain light up when the unpleasant odor is being experienced (Villemure et al. 2006). Diverting the person's attention from the pain so that it feels less painful, that is, being distracted, can be tracked on an fMRI, which shows reduced activity in the brain areas that were brightly lit when the pain was experienced without a distraction.

But before you rush off to ask your doctor to order an fMRI to prove to your insurer that your pain is "real," you need to know that at the time this was written, these tests were available only for research. Also this finding could become controversial. That is, when the fMRIs demonstrate that the dulling of the areas associated with pain takes place because of the patient becoming distracted—the insurer might argue that returning to work would provide the necessary distraction for that patient. In fact, among our patients who are lucky enough to be able to work in spite of their pain, that's often what they report.

body memory: what is it?

Most people believe children before the age of two don't remember anything that happens to them and that emotionally painful experiences during infancy have no lasting impact. Such beliefs might be considered reassuring if they didn't imply that infants also don't remember the love they are given. Does receiving love in infancy have a lasting impact? It most certainly does! As science continues to provide insights into the mysteries of the brain and the nature of memory, we are learning that every emotionally meaningful experience is stored in memory and has a lasting impact on a baby's developing nervous system. And we "remember" a lot more than we realize.

As previously described, the amygdala processes highly charged emotions, and the hippocampus processes narrative or chronological memory. The amygdala is fully developed at birth, so babies are able to feel a range of intense emotions, even though they cannot understand the content of the emotion and its relation to what is going on around them. On the other hand, the hippocampus doesn't fully develop until sometime between the toddler's second and fourth year. Until then, toddlers are relatively unable to organize memory meaningfully in terms of the sequences of events.

It's likely you are aware of the classifications short- and long-term memory, but do you know there are also two other qualities of memory: explicit and implicit? *Explicit memory* is the kind of conscious memory that enables us to tell a story that makes sense of what happened. It reaches maturity at around three years of age. *Implicit memory*, which is available from birth or even earlier, is unconscious and is encoded in emotional, sensory, and visceral recall. In other words, what we don't remember with our minds, we remember with our bodies, with our hearts and our "guts," with lasting implications for our thinking, feeling, and behavior.

If you are unlucky enough to face a situation full of panic or terror from which you feel helpless to escape, the brain sometimes secretes *endogenous opioids* (among which are the endorphins), just as it would in a traumatic physically painful situation, to numb you to overwhelming emotional pain. These endorphins also interfere with your storage of explicit memory, although implicit memory of the trauma can remain available. Experiences that are emotionally too overwhelming to deal with are often stored somatically; that is, as a body memory.

When you forget a trauma, that is simply a defense mechanism, rubbing out your conscious recall. However, the memory of the trauma can be expressed as an unconscious response to stress. Overreacting to mildly stressful or even innocuous situations without understanding why you reacted that way might be the result of implicit traumatic memories dating back to your childhood or infancy. Some of these memories can become conscious through meditation, which although difficult to deal with when they first surface, may provide the opportunity to first emotionally and then physically, heal. If that happens, you may need the help of a therapist.

There is a growing understanding that traumatic events in early life can contribute to the reason that so many people suffer chronic pain. Long-forgotten emotional pain, or pain not stored in the conscious mind, is thought to exacerbate the site of damage in the body and thus prevent healing. For example, despite being in a coma, one man experienced physiological anxiety states when exposed to a smell that was associated with a personal trauma (Grzesiak 2003).

Your brain has an amazing capacity to make associations. Something or someone that "reminds" you of a traumatic situation—a smell, a song, a person who looks like someone from your past—all trigger your automatic self-protective fight, flight, or freeze responses. This reflex reaction can occur too quickly, before the information reaches the cortex where it can be evaluated rationally. That's why you might sometimes overreact to things, people or situations that are reminiscent of a traumatic event, without any conscious recollection of the event on your part.

But even if not consciously remembered, early memories sometimes show themselves indirectly through behavior. It is intrinsically human to reenact defensive reactions to forgotten traumas, even though your reaction may be no longer be warranted. Often, early memories become evident only through persistent feelings that don't seem related to a present situation, or through bodily sensations that don't seem to make any sense. More commonly, early memories of emotional pain or hurt are indirectly evident by persistent difficulties in relationships, particularly in intimate relations.

Implicit memory—or body memory—explains why a woman who was molested as a child remains fearful of intimacy, at least with men who "remind" her of the perpetrator, even though she has not even a trace of conscious memory of the traumatic episode. A man may fear being alone at night because solitude triggers an emotional memory of terror when as an infant he cried in his crib, and no one came to comfort him. He has no recollection of the event, and everyone he knows finds him likeable and congenial. He has no understanding of his compulsive need to avoid solitude. Although successful and fully functional, many people can be avoidant, clingy, or insensitive in their personal relationships due to early traumas, which they do not remember.

These are just some of the relationship problems that have their roots in hurts you might have felt at the beginning of your life. To a greater or lesser extent, most of us suffer from some behavioral manifestations of painful implicit memories.

A Body Memory of a Long-Forgotten Pain

Sixty-year-old Frieda came to our pain clinic complaining of pain in the tops of her feet and in her knees. The pain had come on gradually many years ago and was sometimes intense. We discovered that between the ages of four until she was well into her teens, her mother, who clearly suffered from a mental illness, had disciplined Frieda by having her kneel by her bedside all night. The pain she complained of seemed very likely to be a body memory of those early punishments.

the placebo effect is real

If you believe something is going to take your pain away, it's likely it will: hence a mother kissing her child's painful knee after a fall really soothes the pain. Let's take a look at how your mind functions in its response to pain.

The Placebo Response

Quite fascinating insights into the placebo response have been emerging in the last few years. A *placebo* is a substance or procedure that looks like an active drug or procedure but the placebo itself is not active. In clinical trials for new drugs, pharmaceutical companies test them against placebos, where the subjects testing the drug don't know whether they are receiving the real thing or an identical pill that contains an inactive inert substance. This is administered to test the new drug's effects; however, because the response to the inactive substance can be so high (the placebo effect) it may look as though the new drug is effective, when it might actually not be.

The placebo response has been elucidated by many researchers over the last two decades (Levine and Gordon 1984; Amanzio and Benedetti 1999; Guess et al. 2002). Professor Fabrizio Benedetti described the following experiment at a world pain conference in San Diego in 2002 (Benedetti et al. 2002). A subject was set up attached to intravenous lines (IVs). The pain used in the experiment was created by constricting the blood supply in the subject's arm for as long as the subject could tolerate the constriction. A shot of morphine was delivered through the IV line from outside the room, when the subject did not know it was being administered. This allowed him to tolerate the constriction longer than when no shot was given, *but not for as long* as when a health care worker walked into the room and was seen to administer it. Similarly, a saltwater placebo shot was given through the IV from outside the room and it had no effect; however, it did have an effect when it was given in full view.

So the context of being given the medication is important: seeing the shot administered makes a difference. And even more fascinating, the pain relief the placebo saltwater shot gave was nullified by giving the subject a shot of a morphine-reversing agent called *naloxone*. It seems that it's our own internal "morphine," the endorphins, that are responsible for the pain relief that was felt.

In research done in the early 1980s, patients who had just had a third molar tooth extracted were given a placebo saline shot in full view, in conjunction with the suggestion that they had just received a potent painkiller. It proved to be as effective as a hidden shot of 6 to 8 mg of morphine that was administered without their knowledge. The saline shot gave as much pain relief as the morphine had (Levine and Gordon 1984).

We're conditioned to think of pills and shots as being helpful, so we anticipate their benefits. By doing this, we manufacture the internal chemicals that mimic those being given in the active drug.

Pain and the Anticipation of Pain

Anticipation is a very important aspect of experiencing pain. We've known for years that the power of anticipation is extremely strong. That is, if you want something to work, more often than not, it will (Benedetti 2007). The reverse is also true.

If you anticipate a possibly painful event is going to be very painful, even if only a mild pain is inflicted, it will feel more intense; and if an fMRI scan were being done at the same time, it would most likely light up brightly, correlating with intense pain. Similarly, if you believe a certain treatment will work, it is more likely that it will. For example, a study that looked at the outcomes of acupuncture treatments showed that those who anticipated it would work had better outcomes than those who thought it would not work (Linde et al. 2007).

Thinking the Pain Away

Today, studies are showing that just as you can increase the perception of pain by anticipating it, so, too, you can decrease it—if taught how.

To understand this, you need to know a bit more about how your internal opioids, the endorphins, reduce your pain. In 2001, Jon-Kar Zubieta and his colleagues, used sophisticated imaging technology like fMRIs and PET (positron emission tomography) scanners, to track production of *internal* opioids (endorphins). They watched as experimental subjects produced their own endorphins in their brains while their pain intensities were dropping, after being given a slow painful injection into their jaw muscles.

The endorphins sat on opioid *receptors* that are distributed throughout the brain, like a lock (receptor) and key (endorphin) arrangement, effectively turning down the subjects' perception of pain. The images show a lighting up of specific areas of the brain involved in pain, areas that are known to be sited in the parts of the brain that are involved in perceiving the sensation of pain, and other areas that are involved in the *emotion* that pain causes. The same subjects were given nonpainful injections to provide a control situation that showed less lighting up of these areas.

The experiment's subjects varied widely in how many opioid receptors they had, and in the quantity of endorphins they produced; but the more their brain areas lit up, the lower the intensity of the pain they reported feeling. Both emotional and sensory areas contributed to their reporting of lowered pain intensity.

The same study found that women responded better with endorphin-release when their estrogen levels were high and they were in the later part of their menstrual cycle, which was more in line with male responses.

Zubieta's group (2003) was also one of the first to describe the COMT gene, variants of which are associated with how sensitive you are to pain. This established a genetic basis as to whether you are stoical or more sensitive to pain. It's not all courage!

Researchers at the Pain Management Center at Stanford University's School of Medicine (DeCharms et al. 2005) studied patients with chronic pain under fMRI scanners. The patients were shown how areas of their brain responded to pain by lighting up. The researchers found that those who used mental strategies to decrease their pain were able to reduce it by as much as two-thirds, by focusing on distracting or soothing thoughts.

Changing your mood with pleasant scents also lowers the perception of pain and this correlates on fMRI scans, as shown by Catherine Bushnell and colleagues (Villemure, Slotnick, and Bushnell 2003) at McGill University, Montreal. So we're guessing that shopping for clothes, which produces a serotonin surge in women, likely acts as a pain reliever too.

At the University of Texas, Robert Gatchel, a clinical professor of pain management, says that the brain can prioritize what it attends to, such as when focusing on some other activity like music, a video game, or the breath during meditation. This can create a sort of mental traffic jam which can reduce the suffering from pain (Turk and Gatchel 2002).

emotions and pain—again

All of these sophisticated studies have proved that physical pain is a combination of the physical sensation and the emotion and thoughts it generates. In turn, as adverse emotion builds, it can fuel a greater pain intensity. Quite simply, you can increase your perception of your pain by feeling fear and dread or even smelling something bad. You can decrease it with laughter, pleasant smells, meditation, medication (sometimes in the short term only), guided imagery, biofeedback, and other strategies. Yet the damage visible on your MRI of the painful part of you will not have changed in appearance.

In the next chapter we'll teach you the body scan, where you'll get a chance to put some of what you just learned about pain and the mind into practice.

Chapter 7

reclaiming the parts that hurt: the body scan

Know thyself.

—Oracle of Delphi

You are becoming more aware of your own body and mind and getting new insights just from watching what's happening within and around you. Is your judging of good versus bad turning to simply describing the situation a bit more often than it did in the past? If that's true, how does that feel? Do you notice yourself becoming progressively less tense as you approach the world in this new nonjudgmental way? We hope so, because in this chapter you're going to apply this approach even more intensely to your own body and mind.

Have you noticed how much safer you can feel when you're more in the moment, and how much less likely you are to overstretch or overdo anything because you "weren't thinking?" Now when you note you hurt after doing a certain amount of activity, you are aware you can describe it instead of getting upset over it, and you take a break without feeling resentful.

Your old refrain, "I used to be able to do this with no problem and now I can't," is less likely to be given the same amount of emotional, energy-sapping room in your mind than before. Now it's just a fact that you can't do what you used to do—and that fact doesn't carry an emotional charge. It's just a fact. Taking a break, recharging, and doing a bit more later works better. Little by little, you're taking on a bit more of the "A" word: acceptance. Paradoxically, it's likely you'll find that pacing yourself without resentment or frustration actually increases your capabilities over time. Your energy isn't being depleted by negativity and that energy can be put to better use.

If your condition is a result of an accident or illness rather than simply the normal losses that accompany aging, you might note that being unable or less able to do a task you could do before you developed chronic pain causes more suffering. The unexpected, or undeserved, is always harder to bear than the expected. Similarly, if you'd hated your job and had hoped to retire early, you might be just as upset about being disabled by an accident, injury or illness—which prevents you from working—just as much as if you had really liked your job. The point is this: you wanted the choice. You didn't want it to be imposed on you. Retiring or quitting work voluntarily causes less suffering than being forced to stop working.

Furthermore, if you were getting resentful, you also may have extended that emotion to the part or parts of your body which have let you down and "caused this mess." So acknowledging every part of your mind and body in the body scan and mindful movement meditations is important for taking back ownership of your damaged or poorly functioning parts of yourself, and maximizing what you can do while accepting what you can't.

preparing for the body scan

This meditation brings mindfulness to your own body in all its glory *and* disarray. When you do the body scan, it is as appropriate for acknowledging emotional pain as it is for physical pain, which always contains elements of emotional pain. It's best to do this meditation when your pain is at a lower intensity and to set aside about twenty to thirty minutes to do it. You may choose to lie on a pad on the floor, or on your bed or couch. Or you can sit in a chair, or lie on the floor with your feet up on a chair seat in front of you. You can even stand if your pain condition requires it. Your eyes can be softly shut and your hands gently resting beside you if you are lying down; if sitting, your hands can be resting gently on top of your knees.

The body scan meditation takes you slowly through your body while your mind gently becomes aware of and acknowledges each part, and its function, whether it's functioning as you would like it to, or not. This is not a relaxation exercise. We're not asking you to do anything with each part of your body. You only bring your awareness to each body part just to be present with it, to feel it as it is. You might want to use your own voice or that of a friend to, in a very slow way, tape-record the instructions over a period of twenty or thirty minutes to guide you though this scan, or you can purchase our version through www.painspeaking.com.

Body Scan

Giving yourself over to your breath

Focusing on that to start off with

Breathing in

Breathing out.

And when you've settled,

Becoming aware of your left foot

And the toes of your left foot, noting any sensation in your toes, any pain or discomfort, observing, not judging.

And then the foot itself

*The top of the foot, the sole of the foot
which places itself on the floor*

giving you the support you need, working with your other foot to get you to the places that you need to be.

Even if you have feet that don't work the way you would like, that have been injured in some way, honoring the Time they were working well, and being with them as they are right now, in this moment.

And then becoming aware of the heel of your left foot, up to the ankle and the many small bones that are inside your ankle and allow it to perform so many movements that are important

To allow you to walk, to run, to swivel

Bringing awareness to any and all sensations in the ankle, noticing any intensity or discomfort.

And then going further up the leg toward the shin

The area just under your knee

Aware of the stresses and strains on your knee that occur every day

The muscular tightening in muscles above and below it

And if this is an area for you that is painful,

Acknowledging that it is still an important part of your body, which maintained its mobility for so many years

An amazing joint, carrying so much weight.

Appreciating the complexity of the movement

That the leg does every day, getting you where you need to be and

Working constantly, the lower leg in conjunction with the upper leg, and

Then through the hip, with the rest of the body.

Then becoming aware of the thigh and hip joint

Structures that support you.

And the buttocks, and genital regions

Acknowledging pain, soreness, or any sensations in these areas of the body.

Then around the circumference of the abdomen

From the front to the back and around again to the front

Aware of those structures that are inside the abdomen

Amazing organs inside the abdomen

The bowels, bladder, genital system, liver

Pancreas, kidneys: complex organs working together every day, to enable us to function as human beings.

It's not hard to acknowledge that if not feeling emotionally okay, things can go wrong in some of these organs,

But if feeling okay, these organs work so much better.

Acknowledging the spine, the tailbone, lower back connecting with the upper back

Responsible for so many complex movements: swiveling, bending

For carrying sometimes heavy weights.

But prone to wear and tear, degenerations of time and prolonged use

Still honoring the spine for what it does.

And above the waist

The chest

Bringing awareness to what is inside the chest

The lungs

That are so important for every breath taken

Providing the focus for many of your meditations That life force that we call the breath.

Lungs filled with tiny, tiny tubules In which the air circulates

Through which air diffuses into that liquid we call blood, which allows every organ in the body to be nourished

Acknowledging that blood is carrying oxygen

Through the heart

To be pumped to every organ in your body. Every organ needing oxygen.

The heart: an amazingly complex organ

Not being afraid of it

In fact, marveling at it

Thankful

That long before there was so much technology

There was this amazing organ, which allowed us to develop into living beings

Full of this incredibly complex life.

*Then bringing awareness to your shoulder,
and upper and
lower arm, and hand*

Dwelling within these structures for a while, Then your neck

Aware that inside of it exist those important tubes

For taking air to your lungs

And for taking food

To your stomach

Each nourishing in different ways One nourishing with oxygen

And the other nourishing with nutrients

Both important avenues for allowing the organs of your body

To be nourished to sustain life.

*Then bringing awareness to your face, giving us our uniqueness
allowing us to communicate with other human beings.*

*Mouth, nose, cheeks, eyes, eyebrows,
forehead, hair, ears,*

Incredible, timeless structures

There for us from the first time we were formed

In the womb

Each part of the face

Taking part in our expressions.

Then becoming aware of

*The other side of the body: the right shoulder and arm. And just for this
moment acknowledging your hand
that allows you to pick things up*

To move things

To gesture

Or make intricate movements.

*Regarding your hands in your mind's eye with curiosity
marveling at their complexity.*

And now becoming aware of your upper body down toward the waist.

Remembering again

*To acknowledge the spine And then around inside the abdomen,
acknowledging its organs and their capabilities.*

Bringing your awareness to the right leg

Valuing the muscles: their strengths and weaknesses

They may be a source of pain or discomfort

Of aching, or inflammation, or throbbing

But still marveling at and appreciating them.

Down past the right knee

Into the right lower leg and ankle

With its many bones and tendons. And into the right foot

That part of us that, with our other foot, grounds us to the floor

Enabling us to live our lives

To connect us to people and to other places

And to find nourishment for our minds and bodies.

But every part of our bodies and minds also depends

On another very important organ: our brain

Which controls

Everything you have just scanned

Which makes us into human beings.

The brain providing that center

That tells every part of us

Where it should be in space

What to do

That sends out chemicals

Very suddenly sometimes

Giving us the feelings we have

Instructing parts of our bodies how to move

Sending messages to internal organs

On what chemicals they need to secrete

A power center of our body,

Needing nurturing and care,

Though when we are under stress

It is not hard to imagine

That some of those messages may go wrong

And that parts of the body

May not function the way we wish them to.

And now bringing awareness to the skin

The largest organ of the body

Which contributes to making us unique

Marveling at this structure

Which is waterproof

Such a complex structure which looks so simple

Which provides us with protection and encloses everything within us.

This body scan

Is really a nourishment for every part of us

Celebrating our uniqueness

And ability to nurture ourselves.

Breathing, acknowledging you have taken time just for yourself

The gift of time,

But that by taking this time to bring awareness to your body and mind,

You may do what you have to do

More competently and with an uncluttered mind

For the rest of your day.

When you begin to practice the body scan, you may encounter some of the following common challenges.

Intensifying Pain

Don't be dismayed if you find it hard to focus on the parts of the body that give you pain. This is a common reaction when first becoming acquainted with the body scan. Up until now you may have mentally shunned those parts that you feel have let you down. Sometimes focusing your mind on a painful body part might intensify your pain, but in fact, it is the stress reaction of your mind responding to the pain with a negative emotion. This is a great illustration of how psychological processes can intensify pain. Remember, if we anticipate something bad will happen, it likely will.

This is a splendid meditation for bringing awareness to what your mind does, noticing your adverse emotions, and for practicing being nonjudgmental about the part of your body that has become less able. Acknowledging that focusing on your painful areas brings up difficult emotions is important in the transition to improve your pain management skills. But after practicing for a while, you may be astonished to find that when you bring your awareness to your painful body parts during the body scan, your pain has decreased.

Monkey Mind and Falling Asleep

You may have noticed your mind wandering or perhaps you fell into a light sleep when your mind arrived at certain parts of your body, particularly the most painful or disabled part(s); this can be part of the mental shunning of that part of the body process. Sometimes you can see it's a subconscious defense mechanism. Persistently falling asleep despite lots of practice might be solved best by never lying down for the body scan. Instead, try sitting or standing or slow walking while you concentrate on your different body parts.

Flashbacks and Anxiety

If you have flashbacks to painful memories during this meditation or you have a tendency to panic or you notice agitation, you might prefer to walk back and forth or do a mix of sitting and walking while still going through the body scan. If you uncover a body memory associated with past abuse, always bear in mind you may need to see a therapist. Many participants in our classes were exposed to abusive or challenging situations in their younger years.

Impatience and Dislike

Is doing the body scan too slow? Too boring? Is your life on too fast a track? Are you impatient at not getting to all the tasks you could be doing instead? Remember, doing this once a day for a while can make you more efficient and your mind clearer. So it's worth the time invested. In time, the body scan may become your favorite meditation; the one you'll use over and over again. You may begin to feel awed by how your body works. Or you may not like this meditation and prefer to return to the breath meditations. You may dislike it now, especially if you feel forced to acknowledge a part of your body that you avoid and you can't practice being nonjudgmental yet, but you may return to it another time and find it much easier to do then. Perhaps using the alternative meditations focusing on becoming aware of your adverse emotions over time will enable you to return to the body scan with a new ability to take a fresh look at your challenged body part(s) later.

Cheryl

Cheryl, a pleasant woman in her thirties, was referred to our clinic by a Toronto rehabilitation facility where she'd been an inpatient since a surgery she'd had to her neck a few months earlier. She'd suffered with bad headaches for a few years and an unpleasant pain in her arm and, eventually, a group of malformed blood vessels close to the spine in her neck was found with an MRI, and surgically removed. The surgery left her with the loss of all sensation below her midchest and she had to learn how to walk again while coping with this new strange numbness. The first time I saw her she was in a wheelchair. Her story was heartrending.

One month after surgery, during which time she'd had little pain, a new type of severe headache had appeared. The headache was now constant and much of the time she was in agony. She was given tricyclic antidepressant drugs for pain but they did nothing to relieve it. An anticonvulsant was also given to her for pain but she kept falling asleep while on it, and suspected that it, too, did nothing to relieve her pain. Currently, she was taking sustained-release morphine with some short-acting morphine for an emergency rescue, but they only took the edge off her pain. Two more neurology consultations did not add any new information to help us, and she'd had all the appropriate scans done. We were on our own with her pain.

We worked through the other opioid options and eventually found that sustained-release oxycodone (OxyContin) seemed the best maintenance drug for her and hydromorphone (Dilaudid) the best emergency rescue drug. But when she arrived for her appointments every two to three months, she reported that her pain had been under control for only about one month after the last appointment, when we'd usually had to increase her dose. And she reported that lately her pain was out of control again. Her husband and children were feeling so much stress from watching her suffering the pressure.

As the months passed, changing her medication continued to bring only temporary success. Her doses climbed as we tried to keep her pain under control. We had to give her a stimulant to keep her from falling asleep so often. It was hard on her kids to see their Mom so sleepy all the time. Eventually, she came down with pneumonia, most likely due to her high doses of narcotics, and was admitted to the hospital. Upon her discharge from the hospital, she was placed on permanent oxygen, so she had to use an oxygen tank and a walker, and be confined to a wheelchair for longer trips. A community program paid for an attendant to help her.

So with all of these physical issues to deal with, it was not surprising that she met our suggestion of doing the mindfulness course with a lukewarm reception.

She was set up to take the course at her home via telemedicine from the nearest site. She joined the same class that Derek was in (see chapter 3).

During the course, her preferred meditation became the body scan, even though she could not feel most of her body. By acknowledging her body's separate parts, she began "owning" it again. For the first time her medication needs stabilized. She no longer felt that the medication was losing its effect. She signed up for a second course. Halfway through the course, the hissing sound of her oxygen tank was no longer heard—but Cheryl was present. She was the first patient on our clinic list the next day and we couldn't wait to see her.

She arrived with a cane and without her walker and she was very different. No oxygen, very alert, and very happy. She'd been inspired by Derek's story and his newfound abilities to stop taking his medication and continue his running. One afternoon during a dental appointment her dentist was having trouble completing a filling. He told her he needed to inject more novacaine into her gum because the procedure was taking longer than he'd thought it would. But this would have taken too much time and delayed her, and she had another appointment to keep. She told him to proceed without adding any extra anesthetic, and that she would meditate instead. It worked!

Over the next few days, she became better at going directly to her breath whenever she felt her pain increase, and she began slowly to decrease her medications and to increase her exercise by walking a little bit further daily. Six weeks later, she had decreased her narcotic medications to about one-fifth of their previous doses. To her amazement she noticed that she had less pain than when she'd been on heavy medication. With what we now know about narcotics possibly causing an increased sensitivity to pain when given long term (hyperalgesia), she may have been getting her internal narcotics—her endorphins and her other internal pain management mechanisms back on track again because of her lowered doses. With the aid of a cane she was walking two kilometers a day. She no longer needed her attendant. Her face was full of life and her family was thrilled: their mom was back! She did the body scan meditation every day.

Three years later, and still on some narcotic medication, she's back in the workforce, much to the astonishment of her company's physicians. The reprieve from the clouded mental state her high doses of drugs had caused also allowed her to end her troubled marriage. She set up as a single mom with one of her two teens living with her. One weekend she was in the ER with her son who was sick. Her ex-husband was present. While with her ex, she noticed that her pain had risen to a 7 out of 10 in intensity. And she noted the pain's intensity dropped when he left.

One Christmas when she'd gone three days without doing the body scan, she noticed her pain level rising from her usual 4 out of 10 to a 6. She immediately got back to her daily routine of meditating: her pain level dropped.

Her life has been transformed by mindfulness.

---

movement meditation

If you are too anxious or too prone to having uncomfortable thoughts, changing to a movement meditation is often helpful. You may even prefer this type of meditation over stationary ones. We know that pain sufferers are often scared of yoga, which requires getting down on the floor, so we've modified our movement meditation to accommodate it being done in a standing or sitting position.

The Pros—the Cons

This might be just the meditation for you, the one that finally shows you the value of meditation. It applies the concept of "falling awake" rather than "falling asleep" and being in the moment with the movements of your body. But when you first start, it's essential not to overreach as too many pain sufferers do when they first sign up for exercise programs. Trust your judgment but don't overstretch.

Also, you may have a difficult time emotionally with this meditation because it can really bring home to you the fact that you've lost some of your physical abilities. But it also provides an opportunity to acknowledge how you feel about that; for example, that your loss doesn't feel good. And you can notice such thoughts too. You don't have to be swept away to helplessness and hopelessness by them. Just hold them in awareness. With practice, it truly does become easier to manage those emotions, and to do more of the movements.

At first, don't try to do movements that you think may cause you a lot of pain afterward. With practice you can do more and, even if you do this meditation only two times a week, your balance will improve. Some of your muscle groups may not have been used much lately. So they may feel strange at first. However, it will be gratifying later after practicing brings these movements back into your life. As the old saying puts it: "Use it or lose it." Like the body scan, this movement meditation offers you another opportunity to take back into your conscious mind again those body parts you've previously shunned. It's another chance to acknowledge that, at this moment, certain body parts of yours don't work or they hurt, although that may not be the case forever. Nonetheless, they are still to be acknowledged and "owned." When you do these movements, acceptance may creep in again and look around with bleary eyes in the newfound light.

Mentally Preparing for Movement Meditation

You can mentally see yourself as able to do a movement, even if right now you can't physically do it. You can prepare your limb or body part to do the movement by visualizing yourself doing it. Imagining that you can move that body part, bend it, and flex it paves the way for you to prepare the neural pathways in your brain for that action.

In a workshop we did with Jon Kabat-Zinn, he said that visualizing the movement is an important first step toward making it happen. Visualizing their movements is key for Olympic athletes to accomplish their daunting physical tasks. Instead of saying, "Oh, I can't do this," imagine yourself doing it. Eventually, the movement may happen on its own: your brain may have to see it as possible before your body can comply.

Mindful Movements

Our mindful movements meditation is composed of yoga movements done from a standing position. If you have a disability and you think that by doing any of these movements you may injure yourself, simply don't do the movement but *imagine* yourself doing it in your mind's eye. If you can't do these movements standing up, understand that some of them can be done from a sitting position. Make sure you select only those movements that are safe for you. Don't feel embarrassed if you are doing them in a group or get angry with yourself if you can't do them all. Just trust yourself that you will make the right choices.

Set aside about ten minutes to do this meditation. It's best to stand beside the back of a chair or close to a wall or table to steady yourself. Or do a modified version from a sitting position if your pain doesn't permit standing for ten minutes. Follow the movement illustrations we've included, doing only those you think you can do. Tune your mind into the muscles you use. Between movements go back to the rest position and to your breath. Hear the sounds around you and note that, even if your eyes are closed during movements which require less balance, you know exactly where a limb is at any one point in time. The mind's ability to keep track of where any body part is at any moment (*proprioception* in clinical language), except when asleep or perhaps in deep meditation, is incredible.

So we start by standing upright

In what we call the mountain pose.

Feet slightly apart

Both arms by your sides

Looking straight ahead

And very slowly and mindfully

Bringing awareness to every movement you make

Taking the left arm and lifting it at a right angle
to the body

And then upward toward the ceiling

Pointing the fingers upward

And looking upward

And reaching up as if you're reaching

For something that is just beyond your reach.

And being with the stretch in the muscles

Alongside the torso and in your arms

As you make this reaching movement

Doing every movement mindfully

Remembering to breathe.

And then slowly and mindfully

Taking the left arm down to hang by your side again

Feeling the blood rush back

Into the fingers, acknowledging every sensation.

And then similarly on the other side

Taking the right arm up

To a right angle to your body

And then up past your head reaching upward

Perhaps pushing the toes of your left foot

Into the ground as you reach up to do this

Reaching as if there was something just a little beyond your reach

Like trying to reach for a bunch of grapes.

And then slowly and mindfully breathing

And then bringing your arm down again

By your side

Feeling the sensation in your fingers

Looking straight ahead as you do this.

And now doing some gentle neck movements

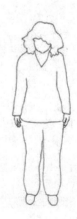

Moving your chin down to your chest

Looking downward and being aware of

The stretch in the muscles in the back of your neck

Remembering to breathe.

And now moving your head in the opposite direction

Now looking up at the ceiling

As you move your head backwards aware of the
        stretch in your muscles

In the front of your neck.

Now taking your head back to

A neutral position

And looking very slowly

From side to side

Moving your chin to your right shoulder

Feeling the stretch on the left side of

Your neck

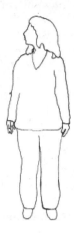

And then slowly swiveling your neck

So that your chin is over your left shoulder

Acknowledging the stretch of the muscles on the

Right side of your neck

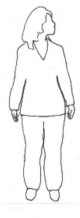

Now slowly move your head back to the neutral
        position

And now leaning your head

Putting your right ear

Over toward your right shoulder

Aware of the stretch in your muscles on the left side
        of your neck.

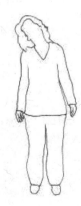

And now moving back in the opposite direction

Taking your left ear

Down over your left shoulder

Aware of the stretch in your muscles

Over on the right side of your neck

Mindfully

Remembering to breathe

And then bringing your head up

To a neutral position again.

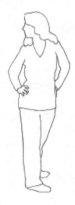

And now placing your hands on your hips

And slowly swiveling

To look behind you

To the right to begin with

Holding that position

Keeping your feet where they are

On the ground.

And then slowly swiveling

And looking behind you

Over your left shoulder this time

Keeping your feet where they are

Mindfully aware of any stretch that's happening

In any of your muscles

And now slowly coming

Back to the neutral position again.

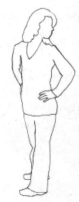

And hanging your hands to the side again

And taking both shoulders

If you can and rotating them forward

Acknowledging the stretch across your back

Across your shoulder blades

As you do this, and

Doing this as slightly or as strongly

As you feel is possible

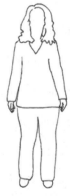

And then slowly reversing the direction

And taking your shoulders and rotating

Them backwards

This time feeling the stretch across

The front of your chest

Mindfully feeling that stretch

And again doing it as little

Or as strongly as you wish.

And now coming back into the mountain pose
again

And now taking the right foot

Placing it about 18 inches from the left

With the foot at a right angle to the left foot

Leaning on that bent knee

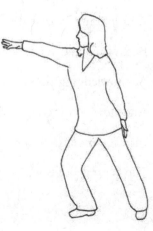

On that right knee

Pointing in that direction

And looking in that direction

And just slowly rocking

On that bent knee as you do this

Only if you can

Just aware of the stretch in the knee.

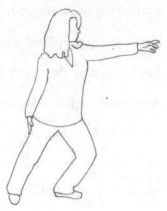

As you do this

Slowly and mindfully

Coming back into the mountain pose again

And changing sides if you can

Taking the left foot

Placing it about 18 inches from the right foot

With the foot at a right angle to the right foot

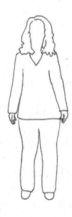

Bending on the left knee rocking to that side

And pointing in that direction with an outstretched arm

And looking in that direction slowing easing yourself

Backwards and forwards onto that bent knee

Acknowledging that stretch in the thigh muscles.

And now coming back again

Into the mountain pose

The central position

Now placing the feet

Slightly further apart

Maybe about 9 inches to a foot apart

And placing the hands on the hips

As we do some hip rotations.

Starting in a clockwise direction

Just rotating the hips

Only if you can.

And if you can't,

Imagining doing this

And just doing it for a few rotations.

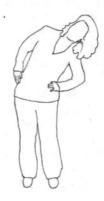

And now reversing the rotations

And going in the counterclockwise direction

Rotating the hips

Gently, as gradually as feels comfortable

Or as much as feels comfortable.

And then just coming back into

The mountain pose again.

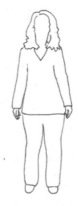

And now first making sure you have a chair back

Available for you, so that if you wobble,

You have something to hold onto.

Just taking the left foot off the floor

Steadying yourself with your arms outstretched

At a right angle to your body

And just rotating at the ankle

As you lift that foot off the floor

Just seeing how steady you are.

And if you're not steady

Just placing the tip of the foot

On the floor to steady yourself

Or just hold the back of the chair in front of you

And just rotating the ankle

And then back on the floor again.

And doing exactly the same

With the right foot.

One foot is often better than the other.

Sometimes you get a little unsteady doing this

But in time your balance improves.

Just rotating your right foot at the ankle

Mindfully

As you steady yourself

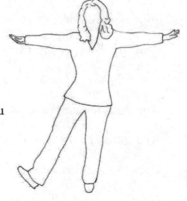

With your arms outstretched

To either side.

And now coming back

To the mountain pose again.

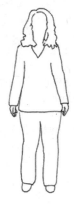

And now taking the palms

Of the fingers

And running the palms of your fingers

Down the front of both thighs

As you slowly and gradually

Bend forwards

Taking the palms of the fingers

Past the knees

A little bit down to the lower legs

And as far as you feel comfortable

And just bending forward

Like a rag doll.

And then just flopping the hands

Toward the floor

And making circular motions with your arms

So that you can see shadows on the floor

Just flopping forward.

Aware of the stretch in the muscles

And remembering to breathe.

And then taking the palms of the fingers, placing
them behind the lower legs

Bringing yourself gradually back up again

As you bring the palms of your fingers up
behind the thighs

Finding yourself standing upright again

With your arms by your sides

Making a little pelvic tilt at the end if you need to.

To just reset things in your spine

Before finishing you might want to incorporate a
period

Of humming meditation, either humming a tune or

Staying at one pitch, taking breaths as you

Run out of oxygen. The hum setting up a vibration
throughout the body

Likely encouraging endorphin release.

Keeping this up for a few minutes, whatever feels comfortable.

And now

Hands on the hips

Taking a deep breath in

And when exhaling

Making a loud noise

As if you are releasing it out of yourself into the room

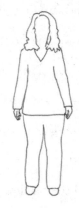

Ahhhh (in breath)

Haaaaa! (out breath)

One more time

Ahhhh (in breath)

Haaaaa! (out breath)

And now you've completed

Your mindful movements.

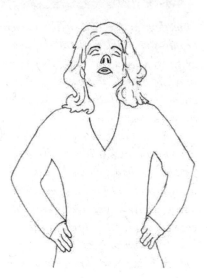

    Maybe you can remember to do these mindful movements every day or a few times a week. Patients report they become more supple, less tense, and have better balance if they do these movements on a regular basis.

    An audio CD of mindful movements can be purchased at www.pain speaking.com.

Anger and Guilt Never Help

One day, at the end of the movement meditation, we noted the class was two people short. Class members reported that one of them had made an abrupt exit, exuding anger, and that another man had gone with him. We found both smoking outside the hospital. When we brought them back inside, the angry one tried, unsuccessfully, to make us feel guilty. He had pushed himself too hard and his neck was hurting badly.

He said that he had to push himself too far because he felt like a "wimp" if he didn't push as hard as he could. Then he became angry. This was the behavioral pattern he had followed far too many times in his life outside class, and it was a huge problem for his long-suffering wife. This gave us the opportunity to point out as gently as possible that his wife's health might suffer as a result of having to cope with his self-destructiveness. He seemed to know about that effect. We said we often saw couples in our hospital elevators and sometimes we wondered if the solicitous caregiver bringing a loved one to our clinic had unconsciously contributed to their loved one's poor health because of their own difficult behaviors. And then, how we wished we could teach stress resilience in the schools to prevent that from happening. Our health system could save a lot of money by funding such programs in the educational system.

We'll be dealing with toxic relationships in chapter 9. But you'll manage the work on that topic better if you've looked after your body and mind first. For now, mindfully reclaiming the damaged parts of yourself as still you— still yours—and beginning to reclaim movements you may not have done for a long time are important.

In chapter 8 we'll look at some ways that can help you take better care of yourself by becoming aware of the physical stressors that influence your health.

reclaiming caring for yourself: your physical needs

Everyone has a doctor in him or her; we just have to help it in its work. The natural healing force within each one of us is the greatest force in getting well. Our food should be our medicine. Our medicine should be our food.

—Hippocrates (460-377 B.C.)

In this chapter we're increasing your awareness of your body and mind's physical needs, starting with the right foods, exercise, and sleep. Just as you wouldn't expect your car to run on low-quality gas, with no maintenance checks, oil refills or transmission flushes, nor would you leave it to stand in the driveway or garage for months to years without moving it, and then expect it to function when you needed it. It's true you could replace it if you found it not functioning by that time—if you could afford it. But you can't do that with your body.

Maybe you could replace certain body parts but not the really key ones. This is the body you will have till the day you die, so it's best to take care of it. It's never too late to start taking proper care of yourself, and it will boost your ability to heal. This, in turn, will make your body less likely to complain to you recurrently with a pain or malfunction or illness "message."

You might say that you'd love to move—if only you didn't hurt; sleep at night—if only you *could* sleep, which is why you catch up during the day, although that never seems to help much. You might say that on your disability income you can't afford good food, and that your spreading girth is due to being unable to exercise because you hurt. And you feel too depressed to monitor what you eat anyway. Or you might say that the prescription drugs you take have caused your appetite to increase. To say nothing about your reduced or absent libido, which makes you feel depressed for your spouse too, which only causes you to eat more.

And with your new moment-to-moment awareness you might notice this self-talk, and ask: Am I really resigned to being this way forever? My muscles are becoming weaker from underuse, which causes my back and joints to hurt more because they have to work so hard without proper support. Do you know that if you put Olympic athletes on complete bed rest for three weeks, they'd be as weak as kittens when they got up? And that, at first, they'd have to take baby steps to gain back what they'd lost? And how long have you been inactive now? One year? Three years? Ten?

Furthermore, it doesn't cost more to eat well—to buy the fuel you need to get your body into shape. If you wouldn't put low-grade gasoline in your car in case it ruined the engine, you haven't got a case for neglecting your own eating habits. You are what you eat. In the British TV program of that name, the dietician host has commented that when the families she works with change their eating habits, they are always astounded to see their food bills go down when they start to eat better.

Sleep is also crucial. A lab rat dies in about nineteen days if sleep-deprived. Moreover it dies of infection. You need to sleep to rejuvenate your mind and body. When you don't get enough sleep or you sleep badly, your immune system is one of the crucial systems to suffer.

You can think of your immune system as somewhat like the police: the lymph nodes are your police stations with their headquarters in your spleen and bone marrow. Think of your fat deposits as doughnut shops (deep-fried carbohydrates, which are changed into fat by your body if your calorie input exceeds your calorie burning): we hope you "get" this analogy. Feed your "police" with good nutrition, give them manageable shifts so they can get a decent night's sleep, keep them circulating briskly, and they will be effectively vigilant and will guard against any threats to your body, such as infection and early cancers. They will also see that your repairs are done in a timely and efficient way.

Simple? Okay, where do you start?

eating mindfully

This is probably the easiest item to start with as it doesn't involve getting off the couch straight away. But it does require a lot of thought.

We know that one medication isn't right for everyone; that is, one person may have dreadful side effects on it and for someone else it's a wonder drug. In the same way, food can have very individual effects. It's important to know the general overview of what is good for most people and then to narrow it down to what really seems to suit you. And we're not talking potato chips and French fries in this chapter. Except, perhaps, as an occasional treat. The rule of 80/20 applies here. The rule states that if you eat well 80 percent of the time, perhaps you can get away with eating less nutritious comfort foods 20 percent of the time.

For another mindful exercise, resolve to prepare and eat a whole meal mindfully. Going out for your meal or getting take-out is also permitted. Every step is to be executed with great attention. The food shopping, the colors, the chopping, the cooking, the table preparation, the smells, and the flavors are all to be experienced mindfully. And for a few hours afterward, note the way you feel. Do you feel too full, too bloated, or just right? Do you feel sleepy or nauseous or sluggish? Is preparing and eating such a meal time-consuming? Yes, so choose a time when you have plenty of time to do it. Is it worth it? Definitely.

Bill Prepares a Meal

Clearly, Bill has never cooked for himself before. A retired pathologist, he likely never connected his work in the lab to the work in a kitchen, but his precision at doing culinary tasks reflects his lifelong commitment to detail in the lab to the benefit of many lives. Clearing his throat he unfolds a couple of pieces of paper and begins to talk to the class.

He speaks of his trip to the supermarket, the wonder of finding out there are so many different cuts of steak, types of lettuce, varieties of tomato, and kinds of dinner rolls. He speaks of the colors, the textures, the feeling of chopping the salad ingredients, the choice of salad bowl, finding the best cooking pan for the steak, and selecting the seasonings. He speaks of the aromas, setting the table, and placing the napkins.

Then he speaks of the steak, the tenderness of the cut he bought (he can afford it, the rest of his class thinks!), and the flavor as he chewed it. Everyone is listen-

ing now, some with eyes closed, smelling the cooking smells as if they were really there, seeing the colors, and tasting the salad and steak. For a few moments their pain takes a back seat to this experience, made all the more poignant by it being so new to the teller. He says that his marriage had been a traditional one. In the past he had never trespassed in the kitchen at dinner time.

He finishes reading his carefully typed pages, folds them meticulously, and puts them into his pocket. Silence. Then someone starts to clap and a ripple of applause goes round the room, although some are surreptitiously thrusting their pieces of paper back in their pockets! He looks abashed. We discuss the role of this exercise in pain perception, and he admits that preparing the meal gave him a renewed appreciation for food.

Paying this much attention to every meal can't be done, but with practice you'll find that you actually notice what you are eating, and you either enjoy it or decide it's not for you. Eat as if your life depends on it—which it does.

And over the next week observe *why* you eat. Do you eat only when hungry? Or when you're bored? Or when you're upset or wanting a pick-me-up, which is why you might choose something sweet, which, unfortunately, would act as a transient, an all-too transient, antidepressant by causing a surge of the brain transmitter, serotonin. Chocolate is the most well-known food for doing that, but a 100 calorie piece eaten mindfully can replace a larger bar eaten mindlessly. You might also find that a 200-calorie cookie can be adequately replaced by a 30-calorie piece of biscotti. You would get the same feeling afterward, but it would be less fattening. Or if you're really lucky, a 50-calorie apple with its beneficial antioxidant properties might satisfy you.

Mindfulness and Weight Loss

Most people have no idea how many calories are in the average muffin bought at the supermarket (about 400 calories for a large one, which is a lot if your daily needs are about 1800 calories), or that sugar is the most addictive substance in the world. A 12-ounce can of soda pop contains about 9 teaspoons (135 calories) of sugar, yet the calorie content reported on the side of the can is only for 100 milliliters (ml) while the entire can contains 350 ml.

Mindful Habits for Eating Right

Now that you're paying attention to food by being mindful, you can take the time to read the labels, understand the caloric contents, and make the right choices. Today, mindfulness courses specifically aimed at weight loss are offered in many cities.

In such a class you would learn that it takes about twenty minutes to feel full after you start eating. So a slower more mindful way of eating gives you greater insight into when it's time to stop. Cleaning your plate isn't something you must do, now that you're not sitting at the dinner table with your mother urging you to eat everything on your plate. That was then—this is now.

At your next meal your new awareness may result in putting less on your plate. Mindfully, you may buy a smaller drink at the ball game and a small popcorn at the movie theater—without the artificial butter. You become aware of the craving you might experience after eating something sweet. If you experience such a craving, you can go to your breath and wait for the craving to pass. The day may come, through mindful practice and observing how addictive sweet foods are, that the rest of the chocolate mousse can stay in the fridge without beckoning you to finish it up every time you enter the kitchen.

Your skeleton has been moving you for a long time but it does age. It is grateful for any help you can give it, especially your knees and lower back. Less weight translates into less wear and tear, which translates into less pain. You may have been on autopilot for too long. Now is the time to be mindful about what and how much you put into your mouth.

Food and Pain

One of our patients with low-back pain observed that she used to eat a lot of foods containing an artificial sweetener and that when she'd eliminated that from her diet, her pain lessened. *Aspartame*, one of the artificial sweeteners, is also commonly associated with triggering migraine headaches.

Migraines and Food

If you're a migraine sufferer, aside from the fact that it is usually familial, it's likely that you've already discovered certain foods are migraine triggers.

A bus driver who took our course realized that he had been taking a peanut butter and banana sandwich to work every day, without knowing that both foods were migraine triggers. He'd been off work for several months, and although he had significant stress in his family, he realized that this was at least a contributing factor to his continual migraines. He returned to work after completing the course, meditates regularly, and has stayed in the work-force more successfully since then.

Migraine food triggers include chocolate, citrus fruits, aged cheeses, red wine, and there are many others. A *trigger* is something that can make you more vulnerable to developing a migraine. However, it may not cause one every time or just by itself. A combination of migraine triggers, not necessarily all food triggers, can make you more vulnerable to developing a migraine headache. Inadequate sleep, sleeping late in the morning, or having a stressful week followed by a relaxed and stress-free weekend, combined with one of your food triggers, can make you much more vulnerable to developing a migraine.

Food, Pain, and Allergy

As you become more aware of your body and mind's responses to food, you may find there are certain foods you really can't eat. It may not be as obvious as a peanut allergy, which can have profound consequences, or a shellfish or other food allergy, which might give you rashes, such as hives. Instead, you may notice abdominal pain, bloating, flatulence, nausea or lethargy after eating certain foods. Take note: those foods might be sabotaging you. You just haven't been giving them your full attention.

Gluten Sensitivity

Celiac disease is an autoimmune disease causing an allergy to *gluten*, which is a protein found in grains in a vast array of foods including breads, cakes, cookies, and on and on. Only a few decades ago, it was thought to be rare and affecting only those who'd first had it in infancy. Today, its incidence is thought to be around 1 in every 100 people in the American population, and the average age of onset is in the forties. It causes bloating, nausea, and loose stool but it also can occur without such obvious symptoms. The allergy to gluten leads to poor absorption of nutrients over all the years the celiac patient goes undetected.

Just as eating a poor diet is a physical stressor for our bodies and minds, this type of malabsorption of important nutrients is also a stressor and can lead to all sorts of problems. Some of those problems are recurrent abdominal pain; osteoporosis, possibly leading to collapsing vertebrae; a greater likelihood of developing depression and behavioral problems; lymphomas; anemia with its fatigue and weakness; and, sometimes, an itchy rash called *dermatitis herpetiformis*. Some people suffering from irritable bowel syndrome (IBS) may, in fact, be undiagnosed celiacs, and can be screened for it by a simple blood test called the IgA tissue transglutaminase antibody.

James Braly and Ron Hoggan in their book *Dangerous Grains* (2002) point out that sensitivity to gluten does not always result in celiac disease, which can lead to the destruction of the absorbing surface of the small bowel. Even without symptoms, sensitivity to gluten can cause the health risks associated with it. Braly and Hoggan list many health conditions, including cancers, where gluten sensitivity is overrepresented in that condition's population, likely was missed in the diagnosis, and likely contributed to developing that condition. In some cases, the condition was reversible or greatly improved by removing gluten from the diet.

One of our patients with Parkinson's disease, a relatively young man in his forties, had recently discovered his shaking was far worse after eating gluten, and he was already eliminating it from his diet. Unfortunately, eliminating gluten before a diagnosis can make the blood test seem normal and can even normalize the intestinal biopsy, which is usually done after a positive blood test confirms the diagnosis. However, his observation applies just to him and is of great value to him. Other Parkinson's sufferers may not be gluten-sensitive but he was able to improve his life by being mindful about what he ate.

It's hard to eat a gluten-free diet, but it can be done and done well, and many products and recipes are available now to help you eliminate it from your diet. Even certain restaurants and food chains are taking notice by providing choices and booklets to tell their customers what their foods contain. You have to become vigilant at reading the labels on the foods you buy in stores, and to recognize the words that imply hidden gluten. Whoever thought that licorice contains gluten? Well it does. And soy sauce is fermented with wheat, which contains gluten. Sensitivity to gluten is also associated with a higher likelihood of juvenile-onset diabetes, which is also an autoimmune condition, and with lactose intolerance.

Lactose Intolerance

Lactose intolerance is much more common now that it is recognized as ranging from mild to severe, can have an onset at any age, and can even remit after being severe during infancy. Mindfully noting that bloating and nausea occur after eating cereal with regular milk, may clue you into recognizing that you have this condition yourself. In that case, if regular milk in tea or cream in coffee does not cause trouble, you might realize you have a mild lactose intolerance. So mindfully you may make your own diagnosis and determine how strongly you react. If your intolerance to lactose is severe however, there are lots of medications that contain lactose as a filler: beware!

Food, Moods, and Behaviors

We've already discussed the connection between feeling more pain when you are in an angry mood (see introduction). In her book *Food, Teens and Behavior* (1983), Barbara Reed, Ph.D., a probation officer, wrote about the interplay between diet and behavior. She discovered that many of the teens whom she supervised on probation had been eating terrible diets at the time they committed their crimes. They ate diets loaded with trans fats, which have no real nutritional value. Even some healthy foods like milk had triggered unusual behaviors in certain individuals, who clearly had idiosyncratic reactions to those foods. She put these teen offenders on healthy diets, which they had to agree to maintain as a condition of their probation. Then she sat back and watched the teens' improved behaviors transform them into model citizens.

Now that we have so much more information about gluten sensitivity (Braly and Hoggan 2002), we think it is possible that some of these teens may have been undiagnosed celiacs.

Jaimie Oliver, the celebrity British chef, must have known about food influencing behavior when he campaigned to change the contents of school lunches in Britain, as shown in his documentary television series. Determined that his own kids shouldn't suffer at the hands of the school system when they started school, he took on retraining the "dinner ladies" who prepared the highly processed foods for their fussy young customers' lunches. He had quite a battle—not only because the children resisted—but cooking good food from scratch made extra work for the dinner ladies.

School budgets didn't really cover the cost of nutritious foods, and the absence of nutritional information among parents all conspired against him. Eventually, his persistence paid off and British school lunch fare is gradually transforming. The ability of the kids to concentrate after lunch is climbing, and in one TV episode, a teacher, who normally provided asthma inhalers to asthmatic kids at lunchtime, reported that inhaler use had been drastically reduced: yes, good nutrition even affects lung function.

The UK is currently introducing mandatory cooking lessons in schools for kids aged eleven to fourteen to learn how to cook nutritious foods from scratch. And beginning in 2008, Quebec has outlawed French fries, soda pop, and junk food from vending machines and cafeterias in its schools. These government actions acknowledge the role food plays in influencing children's concentration abilities; moreover they combat obesity.

The Glycemic Index

We all know that sugary foods can turn some kids into attention deficit disorder look-alikes. The *glycemic index*, which refers to how rapidly each type of food causes a rise in blood sugar after being eaten, is probably at play here. Foods with a high glycemic index are those that cause a rapid rise in blood sugar, which then falls just as rapidly about an hour after eating. These extremes in blood sugar levels occur because insulin is produced in too great a quantity by the pancreas trying to respond quickly to push the sugar into the cells and out of the bloodstream, where high levels are dangerous.

If you've ever seen a diabetic in the ER with very low blood sugar, you've seen what that does to mood. The person is aggressive to the point of spoiling for a fight just before passing out. Give such individuals orange juice while they can still swallow, and they revert to being your best friend! To a less drastic extent that happens to you too, and is especially hazardous if you are prone to migraines.

Our migraine patients on narcotics for their pain know that if we see them in the coffee shop buying a large coffee with sugar and a Danish, they should expect war in the coffee shop. If they have to be on narcotics for migraines, they have to do the decent thing and eat properly!

A precipitous fall in your blood sugar level is really bad for you in many ways. When in the low-blood sugar phase, you may feel on edge and argumentive; your ability to pay attention is poor; and you're more likely to pick a fight. None of this is good for any painful condition you might have. The rapid rise of too much insulin causes your body to store more fat. Too much insulin causes you to secrete more of the stress hormone, cortisol, which is likely why you feel on edge.

Combining a food that raises blood sugar level, such as a cereal, with foods that cause a much slower rise in blood sugar, such as almonds, allows the insulin secreted by your pancreas to be released more slowly too. This, in turn, slows up the blood sugar rise from the high glycemic food. So for breakfast, if you combined a high glycemic food, such as cereal, with low glycemic foods, such as nuts and seeds, you'd likely find you're not so hungry in the late morning and you'd have a better mood and greater ability to concentrate later in the day.

Have you noticed that you're more on edge after eating certain foods or after taking certain medications or drinking caffeinated drinks? By practicing mindfulness you may find that you are more aware that some of your moods influence whether you feel more or less pain at those times.

Eating healthily is a major factor in stacking the odds so that your body and mind function better, which will make it easier to cope with your pain.

Mindfulness and Caffeine

The average chronic pain patient is sleep-deprived. You may be trying to compensate for daytime sleepiness by drinking too much coffee. More than two cups a day is likely to cause jitteriness and interfere with your nighttime sleep. It's not uncommon to hear of nine or ten cups of coffee being consumed in order to improve daytime alertness. More restorative sleep is actually the best treatment for being alert.

Gradual reduction of your coffee intake, even if you have been consuming it mostly in the morning, is one way to manage poor sleep. Note that a sudden elimination or a drastic drop in coffee consumption can cause unsettling anxiety, just like withdrawing from any other drug. After your consumption has been greatly reduced, others may not recognize the new you. Your body language may be so much more relaxed after your sleep has improved. And remember, sleep is also good for your immune system, which needs to be in good shape to support the damaged painful parts of your body, even if the damage took place years ago.

Fluids and Pain

Not drinking enough fluid, especially in hot weather, increases the perception of pain in chronic pain sufferers. The occasional liter of fluid administered by IV restores our patients' pain control without having to resort to increasing their pain medication in some cases. This has happened even in the absence of the clinical signs of dehydration (loss of skin elasticity, inadequate urination); nevertheless, insufficient fluid causing the entire body to be too dry is a physical stressor for them. Not enough fluids also exacerbates the constipation so many of our patients suffer from their pain medications.

For example, several shots of morphine did not get Gillian, our patient with a poorly working bowel, back in pain control for the several hours she was in the ER. Her tongue was so dry it was sticking to the roof of her mouth. After she was given a liter of fluid, she rose from her gurney and attended a Bar Mitzvah that evening.

Foods and the Immune System

We are besieged daily with ads for healthy foods and now supermarkets are making them much more available. So we have fewer excuses for not nourishing our bodies with healthy foods. Antioxidants, found in many foods, such as apples, blueberries, guavas, black tea, and dark chocolate, are really good for your immune system. Some studies have linked them with improved proficiency and vigilance of the immune system to guard against cancers (Knight 2000).

Omega-3, a type of fatty acid, which has been proven to be an anti-inflammatory, is important in providing the building blocks for the membranes of your cells (Wada et al. 2007). And many studies have proved the beneficial effects of a vegetable-rich diet on lowering the incidence of colon cancer (Block, Patterson, and Subar 1992).

Vitamins and Pain

Vitamins are also important for people with chronic pain. Some studies have demonstrated the benefits of 400 mg a day of vitamin B_2 (Riboflavin) to prevent migraine headaches (Breen et al. 1998). Lately, vitamin D has been getting a lot of press because in countries that have cold winter seasons, the people are so deficient in this important vitamin. Supplementation with vitamin D has sometimes reduced pain remarkably, and not just because it assists in preventing osteoporosis. Moreover, a correlation has recently been found between vitamin D deficiency and higher opioid doses.

Dr. Michael Hooten, medical director and anesthesiologist at Mayo Comprehensive Pain Rehabilitation Center, Rochester, Minnesota, reported at the American Society of Anesthesiologists' annual meeting in 2007, that more than 25 percent of a chronic pain population attending a pain rehabilitation center were deficient in vitamin D. That group was on almost twice the average opioid dose, and reported poorer health and worse physical functioning compared to those on opioids who were not deficient in vitamin D.

exercise

The obvious benefits of exercise for relieving pain hardly need discussion; however, as a pain sufferer, you are more likely to ask us, how can you possibly exercise? Especially because you hurt a good deal more when you do exercise. Unfortunately, the painkillers or anesthetic procedures that block your pain sometimes mask too many of pain's warning signs—and cause you to overdo it. Then you pay for exercising with incapacitating pain. So you land back on the couch for a long while.

Finding the right balance of exercise to go with medications and medical procedures is not easy. You need just enough pain relief to allow you more movement but not so much that you'll ignore any warnings from your body while exercising. It's not easy but it can be done.

Even migraine sufferers benefit from being in better physical condition. They report that when they maintain a regular exercise regime (Darling 1991; Koseoglu et al. 2003.) they have fewer migraines and those they do have are less intrusive. Getting into better physical condition is also likely to increase your resilience to emotional stressors, which may be why migraine sufferers report fewer migraines when they routinely exercise. And there's lots of evidence for exercise improving outcomes in the management of low-back pain (Liddle, Baxter, and Gracey 2004).

Exercise is the one sure treatment to limit the severity of fibromyalgia's effects. It helps to reduce body stiffness and maintain mobility, which can be a catch-22 situation for those who have severe fibromyalgia, because it causes stiffness and loss of mobility. But using muscles increases their blood flow and therefore their temperature—so they feel less stiff and are less likely to spasm—and using muscles increases their strength. Then the joints these muscles support become less painful.

Exercising also increases endorphins, which are the natural internal pain-killers responsible for runner's high. It doesn't have to mean doing anything too physically vigorous: walking or swimming is fine.

Now that you are becoming more mindful, you are more likely to be aware when you have reached your limit and stop. And more likely to accept that limit without regret. Taking baby steps at first, can include doing the mindful movement meditation described in the chapter 7. If you can manage gentle Hatha yoga, that would be a really good start.

Yoga

There are many types of yoga but Hatha yoga is the type described by Jon Kabat-Zinn in *Full Catastrophe Living* (1991). He includes its practice as a meditation in his mindfulness-based stress reduction program, which he developed in 1979, and which has now spread throughout the world. Elizabeth Gilbert, in her entertaining best-selling book *Eat, Pray, Love* (2006), explains that yoga in Sanskrit is translated as *union*, meaning a union between the body and the mind. She also refers to the many purposes of yoga, including loosening up muscles and tendons in order to prepare the body to maintain yoga positions while meditating for long periods. It is also possible to access spirituality through meditation.

In beautiful prose she says: "Yoga is about self-mastery and the dedicated effort to haul your attention away from your endless brooding over the past and your nonstop worrying about the future so that you can seek, instead, a place of eternal *presence* from which you may regard yourself and your sur-roundings with poise" (p. 121). This is exactly what mindfulness helps you to do. And by moving your body through yoga postures, you can gently reclaim the ability to move again, far more than you may think possible at this moment.

sleep

Knowledge about the functions of sleep is exploding and sleep laboratories are seeing an increasing numbers of referrals. Their referrals are usually overweight people who snore and have a high likelihood of not getting enough oxygen at night. The problematic neck circumference in a male is seventeen inches: above that, a man likely needs to have a sleep study done.

Sleep apnea is a condition in which the sleeper stops breathing for a short time while asleep. It is characterized by poor oxygenation at night, and has been linked to a higher likelihood of heart disease (Caples et al. 2005). But headaches and daytime fatigue due to poor sleep are problems too. At our clinic, we're increasingly referring chronic pain sufferers to sleep labs for study because so many report struggling with sleep problems like daytime fatigue, restless legs in bed, snoring, and disturbing their partners.

Increasing overweight patients' opioid doses puts them at risk, and even underweight or normal weight patients on opioids have shown some sleep apnea problems. Sleep apnea is treated with a mask or nasal prongs attached to a positive airways pressure (CPAP) machine, which delivers a stream of air at night, so that unobstructed breathing can continue if the body forgets to breath deeply enough while sleeping.

We've also seen extreme headaches and an aggressive diabetic *neuropathy* (nerve damage) pain start a few years before sleep apnea was diagnosed, and we've wondered if the apnea led to the severity and disability of these conditions.

Sleep Stages

There are five stages of sleep: stages 1 to 4 and rapid eye movement or REM sleep. An adult's normal nighttime sleep cycles through these stages about every ninety minutes. Stages 1 and 2 are light sleep: it's easy to arouse the sleeper in those stages. Stages 3 and 4 are deeper, slow-wave sleep and rousing the sleeper from those stages is harder to do and the sleeper may be disorientated on waking. It is thought that the immune system repairs the body from the wear and tear of the day in the deeper sleep stages.

REM sleep is more associated with dreaming than the other stages are, and we all need a certain amount of REM to be healthy. In fact, having no REM or too much REM sleep is associated with depression. Antidepressants can change the amount of REM sleep the person taking such medication experiences. In their book *Sleep and Pain* (2007), Gilles Lavigne and his colleagues discuss the increasing number of research studies in the association between sleep and pain. They make it much easier to understand why the body is so poor at functioning and repairing damaged parts when sleep is inadequate in length or depth.

Fibromyalgia patients don't seem to have much, if any, slow-wave activity sleep in their sleep studies, and sometimes these patients recall they were poor sleepers in their pre-fibromyalgia days. Some fibromyalgia sufferers exhibit wave forms called *alpha intrusions* on their sleep analysis printouts, which makes it look like they wake up several times a night. So, the lack of slow-wave sleep or the intrusion of wakefulness is most likely connected to these patients' sore aching muscles and chronic fatigue.

If you report you are having trouble sleeping to your health care provider, there are actions you can take to improve your sleep: these actions are often called *sleep hygiene*. They should be discussed before you try taking sleeping pills or going to a sleep clinic.

Mindfully Observing Sleep Hygiene

Good sleep hygiene addresses the habits and conditions required for ensuring a long and deep enough sleep to promote good health.

Routine bedtimes. It's best to try to aim for going to bed at the same or similar time every night. Your body has a stress-hormone diurnal rhythm that follows the twenty-four-hour cycle of day and night. This stress hormone, cortisol, should be at its highest level in the morning when you want to be alert, and lowest around midnight when you want to be asleep. This is connected to the light/dark cycle of our ancestors who had no access to the artificial light we take for granted. (It's likely these ancestors had better functioning diurnal rhythms than we do.) Shift workers and travelers suffering from jet lag agree that changing bedtimes is very stressful: so much so that you may feel ill for several days after changing work shifts or returning from a country halfway or more around the world.

Note that if you're recovering from a disease or you are in remission from cancer, it doesn't make sense to stack the odds against your immune system by returning to a stressful shift-changing routine at work.

It's also important to try to rise at the same or similar times each morning, even when you did not get a good night's sleep. You might be more likely to get a better sleep the following night than if you sleep late in the morning to compensate for the lost sleep at night.

Eating and drinking. Eating a heavy meal close to bedtime is not advisable: it's likely to keep you awake. Drinking fluids too close to bedtime is also a problem if you're likely to get up during the night to urinate and you have trouble falling back asleep. This is also hazardous if you take sleep medication, which makes you unsteady on rising during the night.

Caffeinated drinks should be avoided close to bedtime. For some people, they should be avoided after twelve noon. For poor sleepers, it's recommended to drink no more than two cups of caffeinated coffee a day, preferably before afternoon. We've seen people become completely transformed after they've tapered off too many cups of coffee a day, and then experienced improved sleep and diminished restlessness. Note that wine and other alcoholic beverages can also keep you awake. And when awake at night, you may note you crave something sweet to boost your serotonin, which is low at night: It is easy to put on weight if you have insomnia.

Cool room. Your body was designed to lower your temperature somewhat during the night when you have much less muscle activity. Although it's important to stay warm, it's also important to breathe cool air. So keep a window open if that can be done.

Exercise. Exercising earlier in the day rather than just before bedtime enhances sleep. As stated above, this may account for some of the benefit that exercise confers on the pain of fibromyalgia, because a sleep deficiency is a major factor in maintaining pain and fatigue.

TV and/or computer use. Watching TV or looking at computer screens has the effect of tricking your brain into thinking it's daylight. So if you have difficulty sleeping, avoid doing this just before bedtime. Watching stressful TV programs, such as murder mysteries is also likely to keep you awake.

Use your bedroom only for sleep and sex. Have you set up your bedroom to be your office, reading room, and work-out station? Then your mind won't associate the bedroom with restful activities. It is best to keep the bedroom exclusively for sleep and sex. If you must read before going to sleep, it's advisable to do that in another room, away from the bedroom, and to choose soothing reading material.

Avoid daytime naps. You may not have slept well the night before but it may be better to increase the time you meditate rather than nap during the day, which may interfere with the following night's sleep. For those who don't have a sleeping problem, power naps of no more than thirty minutes' duration are good, but that's an entirely different situation.

When you can't sleep, get up. It's better not to toss and turn or lie there becoming more and more frustrated, but to get up, leave the room, and do something nonstressful in a subdued light for about ten minutes before returning to bed. This is when meditation, either sitting still or walking, can be very helpful in reducing the chatter of your mind, which will allow you to let go, and will remind you not to strive to fall asleep. The more you strive to sleep, the less you will succeed. Ruminating and worrying are classic sleep deprivers. Mindfulness and meditation really can help to reduce these habits.

Medication. Sleep medications may help you get to sleep temporarily so you can stop worrying about the lack of sleep. If you can then take it from there without needing to continue taking the sleep meds, that can be very useful. But if taken every night, they usually lose their effectiveness after just a few weeks. And if you try to stop taking them, you will most likely experience rebound wakefulness, which sends you right back to taking them again; even though they don't work very well.

Slowly tapering off sleep meds can help to avoid that rebound, but be aware that there are no medications we know of, including the sedative antidepressants and anticonvulsants, that really increase the restorative sleep phases, the sleep you want. Moreover, some medications may even keep you awake: Individuals vary in their responsiveness. Opioid medications may reduce the slow-wave deeper sleep, the very sleep you need for healing your body.

physical stressors

You may have thought of stress as being primarily emotional, but in fact, as you can see from reading this chapter, stressors include physical stresses such as poor diet, too much or too little activity, poor sleep, and environmental weather and temperature changes. Apart from the weather, if your physical stressors are out of balance and you become more aware of them, change will likely occur over several months to years simply through your awareness—

and it will improve how you handle the emotional stressors you encounter, as your life unfolds. If you feel better, that's already a long way to becoming more resilient to stress.

In the chapter 9 we will talk about the most obvious cause of stress. It often winds its way through your life, and exists within your family, circles of friends, among your neighbors and acquaintances, and in your workplace. No one is exempt from this type of stress unless very lucky. We're talking about *people* stress.

The people in your life can keep you well and extend your life or they can make you very sick and shorten your life span. Knowing this and becoming aware of your reactions to others can set the stage for changing for the better. Reducing your stressful feelings can help your healing and reduce your pain.

Chapter 9

people stress

I learned to become an international diplomat by living
in a household with thirty-four relatives.

—Mohandas K. Gandhi.

The only normal people are the ones you don't know
very well.

—Joe Ancis

It is a fact that if you're emotionally stressed, it's harder to heal and cope with pain. In fact, a pain exacerbation can be connected to an emotionally difficult interaction with others just as much as it can be to a physical activity. So in this chapter we'll look at the many ways you are affected by your relationships with all the people in your life.

Gillian

Gillian was a seventy-five-year-old woman who'd had a very long association with our hospital because she had a bowel that just didn't work. This had been going on since her childhood when she'd suffered terrible constipation. Over the decades she'd had various surgeries to her bowel and had been in and out of our emergency room often.

One day, the gastroenterology department referred her to us for pain management. Over the years when we'd looked after her for her pain, she'd used an opioid pain-medication patch, transdermal fentanyl (Duragesic), on her skin to avoid having to put the medication into a bowel that didn't work. She'd also had up to four shots a day of morphine for those times when her pain worsened. Sometimes we'd change her treatment to hydromorphone (Dilaudid) when her system became too used to the morphine and appeared not to respond at all, despite quite high doses. The shots were injected into a special port, which had been created to access her bloodstream directly, as fluids were also administered in that way. When her pain got too far out of control, she'd come into the ER but such trips became less frequent once she started using the pain drugs with our clinic.

During one of her out-of-control pain admissions she was put on a pump that delivered the morphine directly into her bloodstream; a patient-controlled analgesia (PCA) pump. All she had to do was press a button on the pump to demand the next dose. It seemed to be the answer each time she was admitted, so she had the peace of mind of knowing that her pain would be effectively dealt with—once she had the pump set up.

We were never able to get her to attend our pain management classes because she was always too sick. In fact, for half of her clinic appointments with us, only her husband showed up—mostly to give us an update on how she was doing.

When we visited her during one admission, Gillian was lying in her bed actually pain-free, relishing her comfort and obviously attributing it to the pump. But we'd done the math before visiting her hospital room. Since she'd been admitted, during the last twenty-four hours she'd "demanded" only half of the dosage she'd been using daily at home. At home, the morphine shots were also delivered directly into her bloodstream—so there was no difference in the method of delivery, although she did have personal control over the delivery at the hospital. At home, she relied on her husband to draw up the shots even though both of them could give them directly into her port. And she was in much better control of her pain at the hospital, while never pain-free at home.

We became curious. We had noticed at every appointment she'd been able to attend that she seemed very abrupt and annoyed with her husband—who in fact, was her uncomplaining and devoted caregiver at home. In an intuitive flash, we realized that every time her PCA pump was set up, her husband left her in the hands of the hospital staff for a much-needed break. It was his exit that made her more comfortable. His absence, which always coincided with setting up the PCA pump, was responsible for her improved pain control.

We asked her if we were right. Eyes downcast, she agreed with us, and said that he got on her nerves and had done so for years. She said the times he really irritated her were the times that her bowel pain "acted up." In fact, she said she wished she could have left the marriage years ago. She told us she was completely pain-free at that moment. A few minutes later we heard her husband's voice outside her room. She looked at us pitifully, and told us that her pain level was starting to climb.

Later, we spoke to her adult daughter on the phone. Her daughter agreed with her mother's observations, although we both acknowledged that Gillian did indeed have a very abnormal bowel. It was Gillian's weak point, which was easily triggered by her stressful emotions. "They should have split up years ago," the daughter said, but she also believed that her mother was too judgmental to feel alright in a retirement or nursing home at that time. The status quo would have to remain.

Gillian passed away a year later. In their own way she and her husband were two very caring people; they just weren't made for each other.

But we realized that sometimes, perhaps more than sometimes, pain drugs are prescribed and administered for marriage problems or other toxic relationships.

Relationship Stresses

You are not an island: you live in a society. Your relationships with others can make or break you, can help you heal or make you ill. If you were born more stoical than others by virtue of your genetic heritage, and you were taught by your parents or other caregivers to successfully manage your emotions when you were around people who could be perceived as stressors, it's likely that you've been going through life with few disruptions to your body systems. In fact, you might not need to read this book. If you were born quite sensitive because of your genetic heritage, and your caregivers were exemplary role models who showed you how to cope well with stressful people, you might also be okay throughout your life.

But if you were born a highly sensitive person and your caregivers weren't particularly good at coping with stressful people and situations, and you were exposed to a lot of stress during your childhood, you are much more likely to be vulnerable to your body malfunctioning and to be susceptible to chronic pain.

gender differences

Women tend to be both more sociable and more influenced by their relationships than men. So it follows that if social interactions influence pain perception, then in difficult or stressful relationships, women may be more likely to be debilitated by pain than men in difficult or stressful relationships.

A Canadian study (Moulin et al. 2002) reports that the incidence of chronic pain is about 27 percent for males and 31 percent for females, yet 70 percent of the patients attending our university pain clinics and our courses are female. What's that about? Do men respond differently to the experience of pain than women? Does the stereotypical expectation for boys to be more stoical influence how they handle the sensation of pain throughout life? Are women more emotional about pain than men? Furthermore, if emotions are aroused more easily in women, do negative emotions cause pain to feel more intense?

There is research that says yes to all of the above questions (Jackson et al. 2005). The *cold pressor test,* also known as the Hines-Brown test, is an experimental procedure widely used to examine questions about pain. In this test, volunteers are asked to plunge a hand into freezing ice-cold water for two minutes and they are timed to see how long they can keep their hand in the water before it becomes so painful that they must pull it out. In general, men last longer than women at this.

It is thought that this is so because the male of our species exhibits greater *self-efficacy,* which means that before a man puts his hand into the icy water, he feels more confident that he can manage the challenge than a woman feels. However, when men are asked to focus not only on the pain sensation the ice-cold water causes, but also on the emotion it evokes, they withdraw their hands sooner than when they focus only on the sensation. Perhaps it can be said that, in general, women always focus on a pain sensation with more emotion than men.

The Female Brain

Louann Brizendine, MD, the psychiatrist who wrote the book *The Female Brain* (2006), described the research on gender differences, and shed light on why so many more women seek help at our pain clinic than men do. From infancy, females are responsive to others' facial expressions much more than males are, and females learn to measure their own self-worth from others' expressions. Brizendine says that sometime around the eighth week of gestation, the testosterone surge in male fetuses destroys some of the cells in the communication centers of the brain and encourages growth in the areas of the male brain that govern aggression and sex. However, for female fetuses the cells governing the communication and emotion centers continue to grow and flourish.

Women have difficulty tolerating "flat" facial expressions. They strive to create favorable facial expressions in others. So when women pick difficult male partners, you can almost hear them think, "If I just try harder...."

A stressful pattern may be repeated over many years, which may lead to a mind-body breakdown, and is much more likely to occur in those who are highly sensitive. This in turn can lead to low-back pain, rheumatoid arthritis, fibromyalgia, and migraines. Such a break can take place wherever the genetic predisposition is at its weakest. The first onset of such a break usually occurs after the more resilient youthful body has transitioned into the less resilient thirty-five and over age group.

In 2005, Jackson and colleagues reported that interpersonal transactions have a greater influence over women's perception of experimentally induced pain than they do in men. They reported that when women interact with someone who encourages them to express pain-related distress, they feel their pain more intensely, unlike men in the same situation. Both men and women were able to increase their pain tolerance, if coached and encouraged to do so; the women also increased their tolerance more than men, which suggests a higher response to social suggestion exists in females compared to males.

So why are women so much more susceptible to interpersonal interactions with others than men are? Brizendine says that women's very survival depends on these social interactions. Survival of the species depends on women's ability to read their infants' faces accurately to be able to nurture them appropriately. Moreover, because women have less physical strength to flee or to fight, being able to read the face of a potentially dangerous male must have been an important skill throughout human evolution.

Women are less able to engage in the fight-or-flight strategy when pregnant, nursing or caring for a vulnerable child. Consequently, the ability to form social bonds to group together and get the protection of other females is important for survival. Females bonding in groups can help to protect each other from male invaders, a strategy Brizendine refers to as "tend and befriend" (p. 42). She cites a study on female baboons where the females who were the most socially connected had the highest number of surviving offspring.

stressful relationships cause pain

In *Full Catastrophe Living* (1991), Jon Kabat-Zinn describes interactive martial arts exercises, such as those used in aikido and suggests using them to role-play in order to really feel the emotions associated with the behaviors they demonstrate. We suggest you try these with a trusted friend or family member, or with your therapist if you have one. The exercises may help you to identify the behaviors you use most often in your regular interactions with others, and then to feel the behaviors' associated emotions and their influences on your physical pain experiences.

The Aikido Exercises

These exercises always take place between two individuals: an attacker and a victim. Kabat-Zinn describes four sets. It is best to read their descriptions carefully before trying to do the role-play. It is also important to decide whether your physical condition and your opponent's will allow physical role-playing without injury. If you are not able to do this physically, then create a scenario in which you role-play with words only. Words alone can provoke physical pain powerfully, as we all know.

Aikido Exercise 1

In this exercise, the attacker charges forward toward the victim and the victim cowers before the attacker, the picture of submission. The victim tries to do anything to appease the attacker and defuse the situation. Or the victim might "freeze" with fear instead.

Commonly, this scenario evokes feelings of frustration and disgust in the role-playing attacker, and the sense that nothing has been resolved. It also might increase the attacker's tendency toward violence in order to provoke more of a reaction from the victim or to vent frustration.

The role-playing victim may feel temporary relief if the danger passes, but often also feels some suppressed rage at having been put into this position. The victim also fears that an attack may happen again, and may feel self-contempt at being unable to mount any kind of defense.

As a witness to this role-playing exercise, you might feel disgust or pity for the victim and anger toward the attacker. If you recognize some of your own past behavior as an abuse victim, you may become upset at seeing this scenario played out; you might even feel nauseated or fearful, and relive the feelings you had when the abuse occurred. Should this happen, perhaps you also will be able to acknowledge that your entire body has been affected by the associated emotions, and that your physical pain intensified while you watched.

You might also remember being a child who watched this type of interaction between your parents or caregivers. Did you feel angry with the victim for being submissive? Did you identify with the child who felt endangered and vulnerable because the victim couldn't risk protecting you, when you were a child in a similar situation? Perhaps this vulnerability led you to side more with the attacker and to feel disgust for your victimized parent? Angry feelings are easier to bear than helpless hopeless feelings.

If such long-ago situations are brought to mind by the role-play, watch for other physical symptoms that might occur as your body memories are evoked by the scenario. Memories can lead to feelings, which can lead to physical symptoms, such as the exacerbation of pain.

Aikido Exercise 2

In this exercise, the attacker charges at the victim who, at the last moment, triumphantly moves out of the way. As the attacker, you are likely to feel frustrated, angry, and confused at the absence of engagement. As the victim, you may feel temporarily victorious that you avoided the conflict and remained safe. But that emotion may soon be replaced by feelings of sadness, anger or perhaps disgust at having been in that position. As a witness, you might feel relief for the victim and anger toward the attacker, but you may also feel some guilt because this may be a scenario you participated in recurrently for years: that is, avoiding an issue that needed to be addressed.

Aikido Exercise 3

In this exercise, the attacker and victim come at each other and lock in combat, each fighting the other, moving backward and forward like a pair of wrestlers, but neither one is victorious. You might feel this as a much easier emotional experience, with each new feeling strengthened by your anger and adrenaline rush. You may feel a temporary state of euphoria from defending yourself "respectably." At that moment, your physical pain may be at minimum intensity as your endorphins are released. Watching this scenario can also feel okay because you don't see anyone actually diminished, but afterward you note there was no resolution.

In these three exercises, the problem causing the conflict does not get resolved. Nothing changes. Scenarios like these are played out again and again in households and workplaces in countries all over the world. They are a waste of emotional and physical energy and they drain your body's ability to stay balanced and well. Perhaps you can see that constantly replaying conflicts has a bad effect on your body-mind's ability to stay healthy and balanced. Your sleep and health habits may also have been affected by the nonresolution of problems.

Where Does Nagging Fit Here? An interaction in which one person constantly speaks "at" another is just as debilitating as scenarios 1, 2, and 3. The victim may comply grudgingly to keep the peace (aikido exercise 1), appear to not hear (aikido exercise 2), or flare up into a temper and shout back (aikido exercise 3). You may recognize this role-play as a familiar interaction with a spouse or an offspring, particularly a teen. If so, it's time to ask yourself if this type of interaction has been effective and, if it hasn't been effective, to acknowledge that the time is long overdue for you to search for an alternative interaction; one that "works."

Aikido Exercise 4

In this exercise, the attacker first charges at the victim, who then comes toward the attacker and gently but firmly grasps the attacker's wrist, turning both players simultaneously to face the direction in which the attacker is traveling, and sharing the momentum in that direction. The attacker slows, contact is established, and the two slow down and walk together in the same direction.

This is referred to as *blending.* It can be seen as taking the middle way—or perhaps as compromising.

In this scenario if you are the attacker, you might feel confused at first because you and your attack are being *defused,* but contact is made, which is not unpleasant, and you may feel as though you are at least being acknowledged. A partial validation has happened, which is better than none.

If you role-play the victim, you are using the wise mind: blending reasoning with emotion, and staying grounded even in the face of a threat. This scenario takes energy and resolve but it is more satisfying than the other three. And it is more likely to result in resolution, rather than the constant revisiting of a never-resolved problem.

If you witness this interaction, you might note a feeling of relief at not having to witness an unsettling and unresolved conflict. Perhaps you may feel respect for the way the victim handled a potentially difficult situation. You also may realize that some of your previous unproductive responses to threats or challenges might have been changed to this middle-way approach.

Part of the success of taking the middle way lies in its validation of the attacker's perspective, even when that is very different from your perspective. An area of psychology known as dialectical behavioral therapy (DBT) uses this as a strategy, and it can be very effective.

Dialectical Behavioral Therapy (DBT)

This strategy holds that, however difficult it is to see, you may be able to find the attacker's justification for seeing things and behaving in the way that he or she behaves. And when you understand the attacker's justification, you can see how the attacker might feel that way. And then you are seeing the situation in a different way. By partially validating the attacker using this kind of dialectical thinking, which may be a new concept to you, you may find that it is very helpful toward resolving a conflict situation.

Tone of voice. Your voice is very important in this approach. It should not be raised and should be somewhat conversational but not too conciliatory. With practice, you may become aware that the same words you might use in an argument—but spoken in a conversational nonthreatening way—yield a better outcome than the knee-jerk reflexes of shouting, accusing, or making highly anxious statements. "This is easier said than done," you might say. But the consistent practice of mindfulness has certainly helped us "to think before we speak" in our interactions with the teenagers in our families. And that has made a big difference!

Body Language. Mindfulness may help you to note how you physically react adversely to perceived threats and slights, and that others subconsciously sensing your reaction, in turn, respond more problematically, which can increase your physical pain. This can have a ripple effect of making the communication worse. Now, mindfully aware of these habits, in time, old physical responses may change and communications may open in ways you might never have imagined.

dialectical versus dichotomous thinking

To understand dialectical frameworks, you can think of the many apparent opposites we all encounter in daily life. In his book, *Don't Let Your Emotions Run Your Life* (2002), Scott Spradlin explains that dialectical thinking is the understanding that a statement such as, "expressing your emotions is a good thing to do" does not contradict its opposite statement, "controlling your emotions is a good thing to do." Dialectical thinking states that over time, the two statements will synthesize into "expressing and controlling your emotions are both good things to do."

In contrast, *dichotomous thinking* is "all-or-nothing" or "black-or-white" thinking. It's also a kind of trap. On the one hand, you think you should be able to control your emotions. On the other hand, you think you should be able to express your emotions. Which proposition is true? Is one true at the expense of the other? This is a much harder way to live and results in being overly judgmental.

Dialectical thinking is more flexible and replaces the idea that life can only be this or that, with the alternative that life is both this and that. "Or" thinking is replaced by "and" thinking. Dialectical thinking is about finding the middle path between extremes: the extremes of emotion (for example, suppressing emotions versus overreacting), or extremes of thought, especially about relationships (for example, "they either love me or hate me" rather than "they both love and hate me").

When you're confronted with apparent contradictions or conflicts in your life, with help from your mindfulness skills, you may find yourself turning toward tolerance for different opinions. In the case of interpersonal conflicts, letting others set their own personal limits while you set yours, knowing that everyone's limits can fluctuate from time to time and they don't have to be set in stone, becomes far less stressful. Life isn't all or nothing. It's usually both/and.

Managing Difficult People

There are times when it is important to recognize that a dialectical approach will never work because the attacker lacks insight or is unable to negotiate with the attacked person. To be able to let go of needing to be validated or acknowledged as "right" seems to get easier as you become more mindful. This might also involve making choices to limit or eliminate the time you spend with such individuals, or to be like "Teflon" in your interactions with them. That is, nothing they say sticks to you. They can still make their difficult comments or behave in ways that irritate or are disrespectful, but you no longer react to such negativity with an adverse emotion.

You no longer take it personally or take them seriously, and you don't even have to let them know you are doing this: eventually, they may realize that they no longer have an impact on you. The important point is that when you feel this way, they are no longer able to influence your health adversely, and the exacerbations of your pain that were caused by them in the past become muted or eliminated.

Living with Abusers

If you are still living with someone who is abusive, you must recognize how much your health has been destroyed by your proximity to this individual. You may feel too helpless or hopeless, too sleep-deprived, and too ill to think about getting out of your situation, but don't be fooled into thinking that your physical health and your pain are not connected to your emotional situation: They are. Look into abused spouses' organizations, talk honestly to your doctor, get the help you need, although at the same time you must understand that your life won't be great until well after you're clear of this situation. Be careful and as wise as you can be when taking your leave. Plan your departure well: you might need to alert the authorities if you think there could be a threat to your safety during your transition or afterward. Don't give up on your life, on the possibility of ever becoming okay again. No abuser deserves that much power over another individual.

Abusers come from all parts of society and your abuser may even be employed by one of the authorities we just suggested you should approach. Abusers may appear to others in your community as upstanding members of society. Know that you are not alone: we hear about these types of frustration from others in our clinics. Abused spouse organizations can still help you and will suggest ways for you to seek protection and counseling.

Chronic pain, particularly, responds poorly to medications when abuse is active in a relationship in your life. So don't make the mistake of not telling your health care provider that you are abused in case your provider doesn't take your physical pain seriously. Remember, even though your pain is coming from a physically damaged part, it still may become less painful when you make the transition to a calmer and emotionally more comfortable life. Even your allergies can improve.

The "not right" relationship. Interestingly, even when you are not abused but your relationship is just "not right" for you, that too may have an effect on the intensity of your pain.

Jay's Pain

Jay had been away too long. If he had been taking his opioid medication at the prescribed dosage for his severe low-back pain, he should have returned to the clinic for a renewed prescription. In our clinic, opioid medications are renewed every ten to twelve weeks, and we had to see the patient in person for that. Although he had been stable on his dosages and able to work in light occupations, he had a "difficult to watch" edginess and a physical tremor, especially when he was anxious, and there was some question as to whether it was due to his medications, which we'd not seen described in the literature.

One day he arrived at a maintenance meditation class. He just dropped in as he lived two hours away and could not attend regularly. He looked relaxed and happier than we had seen him for years, and he had hardly any tremor.

He shared the news with us that he had separated from his wife and was now living with a new partner, a childhood sweetheart, with whom he was very happy. His back was much less painful and he'd been able, over time, to reduce his medication dosage to a third of what he'd formerly needed. The tension in his back muscles had lessened considerably.

In his marriage he'd lived with his in-laws, and we remembered that when he'd finished the mindfulness course, the only place he'd been able to do his daily meditation was in the garage using his car's CD player. The course had led to his resolve to move with his wife into their own place, but it had not helped his marriage, and they had gone their separate ways. His whole body was now clearly reaping the benefit of his back pain having lost its intensity, and "morphing" into a discomfort, which was far less disabling and more easily treated.

Exercise: Think about the people in your life. Do you associate any of them with pain exacerbations? Do you dread holidays like Christmas, Hanukah, and Thanksgiving because family members will be present you'd rather not see, or you'll be unable to get time alone, which is how you sometimes have to manage your pain and they don't understand? Can you bring beginners mind to these situations, aware of how you have been reacting and responding to them in the past? Remembering the "ripple" effect, they may become aware of the new way you are perceiving them, and respond to you in ways that are far less stressful for you all.

seeing is believing

In chapter 10, we urge you to express your pain on paper by making art. You might want to draw it and color it. You might choose to make models of your pain or to write about it. You might want to use art as a way to depict difficult family situations, which have influenced your health. You don't have to be good at art. Just pick up a pencil or a brush: you'll be surprised at what you come up with. Making art can be a great way to dislodge powerful thoughts or feelings that have been stuck inside of you and need to see the light of day. Making art may allow a whole lot of pain to be released from your body as the artwork unfolds.

Chapter 10

art:
see the pain—feel the gain

Art opens the closets, airs out the cellars and attics. It brings healing.

—Julia Cameron, *The Artist's Way*

In this chapter we hope to inspire you to start expressing your true feelings and emotions through art. You might find this easier by looking at examples created by our patients. Like them, you may find that expressing yourself through art can be a means to increase personal awareness and reconcile conflicts. When dealing with chronic pain, anxiety, high stress, and depression, art can serve as a valuable tool through which one's innermost thoughts and feelings can be expressed. Making art may help you to communicate with others when words can't be found or are inadequate to describe what is really happening.

Emotions have always been a part of experiencing and generating art, as well as part of the experience of pain. Many great works of art were produced under stress, out of depression or frustration, or as the result of an intense need to communicate. The works of Vincent Van Gogh are a strong example of this need. Picasso's *Guernica* is famous for the rage and grief he communicated in the painting, which was painted shortly after the Spanish village of Guernica was bombed during the Spanish Civil War.

You will find that creating art taps into both your conscious and unconscious mind and it may offer you surprising insights into your life. It also will provide you with a representation of your current situation, thus allowing you to review your progress months after your artwork was created. You can use paint, clay, pastels, crayons, or simple pencil and paper. And remember, it's not about showing off personal talent but about accessing the power of your nonverbal images to move your spirit in ways that words alone cannot.

artwork from pain sufferers: some examples

Many chronic pain patients have said that they benefit greatly from seeing the pictures other chronic pain sufferers have drawn and painted. When insights are shared, they help to fuel personal growth and the willingness to look more deeply into their own pain experiences. We are forever grateful to our pain patients for their willingness to graciously share their images about their pain with you in the following pages.

It is often important to share your artwork with others. We hope you will discover in the examples we provide that there are times when other people's input can provide you with insights into your own art. You may find that you did not consciously intend to express something on paper, but your subconscious mind found a way to express itself in addition to your conscious mind's directions. When other people have the opportunity to comment on your art and express what they see in it, that may help you make connections to deeper insights.

Paul

Years ago, Paul was the first patient in our Mindfulness-Based Chronic Pain Management course to use art as a way of expressing himself when he was asked to practice a mindful task. Paul opened our eyes to the healing power of art, paving the way for hundreds of participants in our subsequent courses to benefit similarly. Paul started to create art because of the difficulty he had expressing his feelings about his chronic pain. He felt that his back injury nineteen years earlier had thrown him into an endless world of doctors, surgeries, medications, chronic pain, and difficulties with his insurance company. He also felt that, "Nobody wanted to hear about it anymore" and so he said nothing. Even when he was encouraged to speak about these awful experiences, Paul remained blocked. It was another class participant who suggested that Paul might try to express his feelings through art. Paul went home and immediately started drawing. In the first week he drew fifteen to twenty pictures. In fact, Paul became a prolific artist. He'd finally found a way to express his frustration that he couldn't otherwise "get out on the table."

When Paul first enrolled in our Mindfulness-Based Chronic Pain Management courses four years ago, nineteen years after suffering a catastrophic accident at his job in highway construction, he began to review his life. He had spent years of his life in bed, depressed and dependent on Demerol (meperidine, pethidine). Feeling "invisible" he had chosen to further seclude himself by moving to a remote farm with his family and slept up to fifteen hours a day in bed. Paul's only activities had been going to doctors' appointments and fighting his insurance company for his benefits. In time, Paul's depression gave way to anger which spilled out onto his family causing his wife to pack up the children and leave.

It was during that time alone that Paul began to look deep within himself in what he calls "prayerful meditation." He began to cry at the "images" he saw of himself in his mind. After going through that, he began to feel encouraged that he could finally free himself of his anger, depression, and low self-worth. Paul's wife and children returned home. Meanwhile Paul started to reach out for more contact with others by joining the church choir and volunteering to help run the local boy scout pack.

In 1998, Paul started to receive treatment for his chronic pain in our pain clinic. We helped him to better manage his pain and encouraged him to continue exploring and sharing his thoughts and feelings by joining our classes in meditation. It was there that Paul found a way to describe through art the remarkable pain journey he had been through. Reflecting today, Paul says, "The Mindfulness course helped me to feel heard. It moved me forward in body, mind, and spirit."

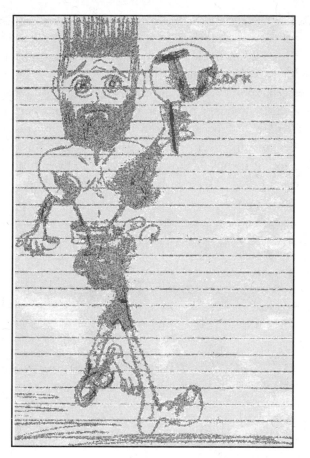

Tied Up in Knots

I used to be so strong and big that my highway construction company worked me like two men. I got a lot of my self-worth through this physical activity. Then I had my accident and I haven't worked since (nineteen years). In my picture, my hair is standing up on end because of fear. Fear because I didn't finish high school and all my value was in my physical strength. The magnifying glass over the word "work" is making work harder to see, to know what the future holds. I'm tied up in knots with pain. My eyes are bloodshot due to lack of sleep. I am exhausted mentally, emotionally, physically. Legs, arms, and back all ache with pain. The turning screw around my waist is where they implanted screws and took bone from a donation site in my hip. The knotted stomach is from an ulcer due to my meds, until I learned that juicing raw cabbage took that pain away.

—Paul L., forty-four
Back Injury Sufferer

Today Paul is struck by the fact that he was so passive. In fact, since injuring his back he had chosen to no longer cut his beard. It was as though he had placed his life on hold, doing nothing, and waiting for his pain to pass before undertaking anything.

Paul's whole outlook began to improve so much that he began to experience "a new sense of hope, peace, and joy." In time, Paul realized that his physical strength had been replaced by a greater inner strength and a newfound ability to work with others. In fact, Paul won an award from the Optimist Club for his involvement with the youth in his community. He feels that the best reward of all, however, has been to reunite emotionally with his wife and family.

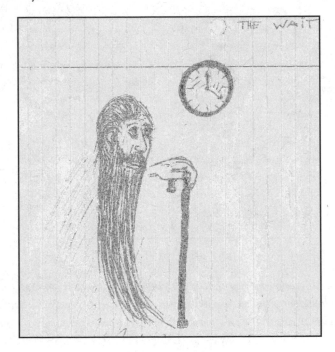

The Waiting Game

When I first got injured, I felt everything in my life was in everyone else's hands: the doctors and insurance company. I stopped living and became a clock-watcher. To mark time, I decided to let my beard grow and it got very long with me waiting. This picture summarizes how I felt having my life on hold, having no power.

—Paul L., forty-four
Back Injury Sufferer

Mike

Mike was born with *hydrocephalus* (water on the brain) for which he'd had three shunts surgically inserted to relieve the fluid buildup in his head. Despite these shunts, Mike says he has never known a life without constant migraines. This next picture, drawn in a minute, is an excellent example of the unconscious mind being expressed through art. The large "boulder," a metaphor for his pain, looks very much like a human brain threatening to snap his brittle body. Interestingly, Mike never made the obvious connection between the boulder and his brain until it was suggested by us.

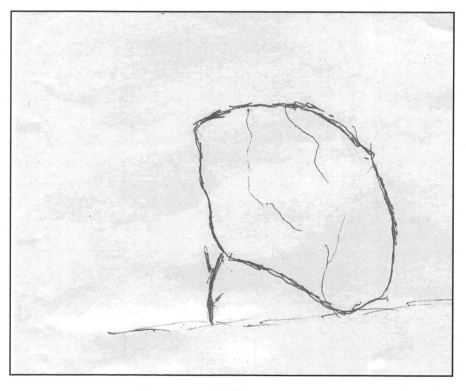

My Pain

The rock represents the pain I feel every day. The twig represents me. The rock is much larger because I find the pain overwhelming.

—Mike S., twenty-four
Migraine Sufferer

Sarah

Sarah grew up in a series of foster homes. She was sexually and physically abused in her last foster placement. After adoption at the age of seven, the abuse continued until she bravely left home at age 15. She has lived with debilitating migraine and spinal injury for many years. Her picture seemed to express her anguish. Originally a dancer and actress, mindfulness allowed her to return to dancing and also deal with the additional burden of the pain of a slow-growing, rare, head and neck cancer. The exaggerated distortion of her face represents the actual distortion that is occurring because of the cancer. She believes she would not have survived until now without the mindfulness programme.

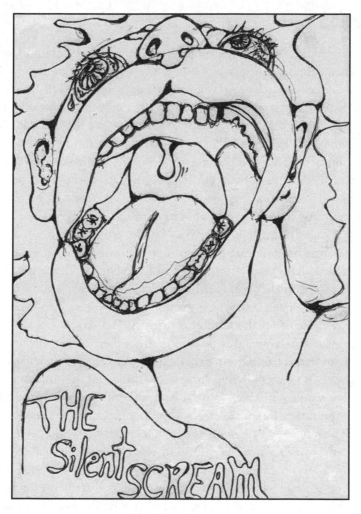

The Silent Scream

I began to draw this picture in the midst of an excruciating migraine. My eyes were bulging with swollen, red blood vessels and tears were streaming down my face. As I finished the picture, my pain diminished. It had gone from a 10 to a 3 out of 10, which is very unusual for me and something I've never been able to recreate. I'm now able to reassure myself in the midst of a severe migraine that the pain will eventually go. Before I started mindfulness classes I could never do that.

—Sarah M., fifty-one
Longtime Survivor of a
Rare Head and Neck Cancer

Martha

An only child, Martha grew up in a prairie household full of adults including a pedophile uncle who abused her under her family's "Christian noses." At sixteen, Martha ran away from home and entered into a succession of failed marriages, eventually marrying her current husband with whom she has two children. Martha's health problems began with the birth of her first child and were exacerbated after the birth of her son five years later. Her husband's business failed, he became an alcoholic, and developed cancer. He later recovered from the cancer, but his psychological scars have been slower to heal. Martha feels that their lives have slowly been getting better over the last ten years, and her ultimate goal is to enroll at a university.

What is significant in her drawing is not only the metaphor that she chose to describe her suffering but also that her husband is facing backwards in the wagon, looking away from the rest of the family. This implies that his depression, rooted in the past, is currently impeding his relationship with his children and his wife. He drags an anchor behind the wagon, which makes it even more difficult for the family to reach their goals.

When Martha showed this picture to the others in her class, there was an immediate flash of recognition that came over some of their faces as they identified with its theme—living with an unwilling and dysfunctional partner. We're left to wonder whether Martha and her children would be better off if they let the father disembark from the wagon. Certainly, her load would be a lot lighter if he were left to stew in the mud. He will choose to either stay there or move ahead, neither decision being something that Martha feels she has any control over, in the final analysis. And in the end, does he resent her for being the one who pulls the wagon thereby disempowering him even further? This is a difficult situation for all, no doubt one that contributes significantly to Martha's pain and suffering.

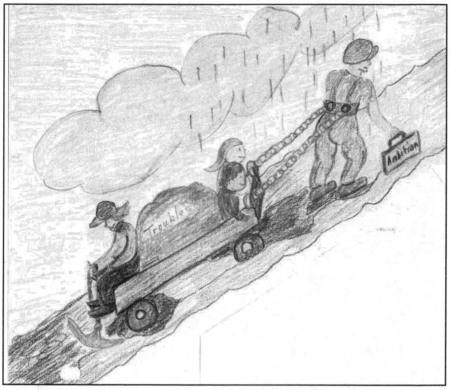

My Overall Mood

The path I have chosen for my journey through life is a steep uphill struggle. The road I am traveling upon is rough and filled with potholes. It is a heavy load to bear but the burden is precious. Therefore, I have willingly chained myself to this wagonload of troubles. The kids are along for a rough ride but have been given the front row seat. I want them to put their troubles behind them and keep their eyes on the road ahead. Anchored in the mud of depression, their father is letting our pack of troubles hold him back and come between himself and our children. The anchor of unemployment means slow and painful progress, but giving up is not an option. My thinking cap is firmly planted on my head and my jaw is firmly set. I have managed to hold onto a significant ambition—higher education. It is raining on my parade. However slow the pace, one small step at a time I plod toward the goal ahead. I am making progress.

—Martha L., fifty-five
Fibromyalgia and Depression
Sufferer

Marie

Marie was one of the most severe fibromyalgia sufferers we ever met. She had only two chairs she could tolerate sitting in: one at her home and one at her psychotherapist's office. She would be in excruciating pain if someone jostled her even slightly when she was out in public, and the noise of the washing machine lid slamming shut could put her into extreme pain for hours afterward. (It was after hearing this from Marie that we realized loud unexpected noises could put us into transient physical pain also.)

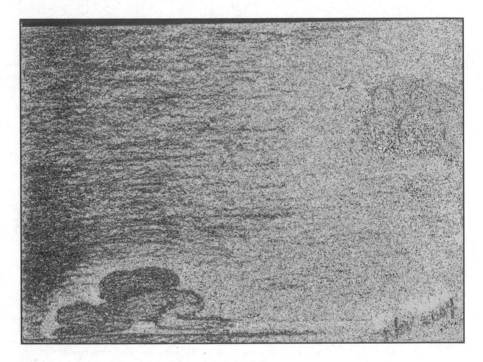

A Year in the Life of My Pain
Picture A

Picture A was made in the first course I ever took. It was an easy picture to draw. It came into my mind in thirty seconds: No hesitations. In it, I'm weighed down by a heavy pack. It's like an albatross around my neck, getting heavier and heavier. I kept all my pain inside, thinking that by avoiding it, it would just go away and by not talking about it, I was being strong. However, I was really misguided because I became more and more depressed over the years.

Actually, I was being a coward, as I have now realized after taking the pain management courses that facing my pain is the most courageous and beneficial thing I have ever done in my life. The darkness in these pictures is overwhelming, all-encompassing, all-consuming, and it tainted every thought, action, emotion I had every day of my life, and I didn't even realize it. It had that much power over me and I didn't even know it. The darkness relates, in part, to religion because I feel evil, bad, unworthy, and that I don't deserve good. Religion, good versus bad, played a large part in my childhood. This is related to things my mother said to me as a child. It also relates to how she interacted with me: withholding love toward me physically (no hugs), verbally (never saying "I love you", never saying "I am proud of you"), and emotionally.

A Year in the Life of My Pain
Picture B

Picture B was drawn in my second course. I felt some people had grown closer (my classmates) because, with them, I had some "light bulb" moments. There is light but it's not all light because everything hasn't been figured out yet. Other people are in the light. I had done talk therapy in the past, but didn't feel the weight lifting off my shoulders with that.

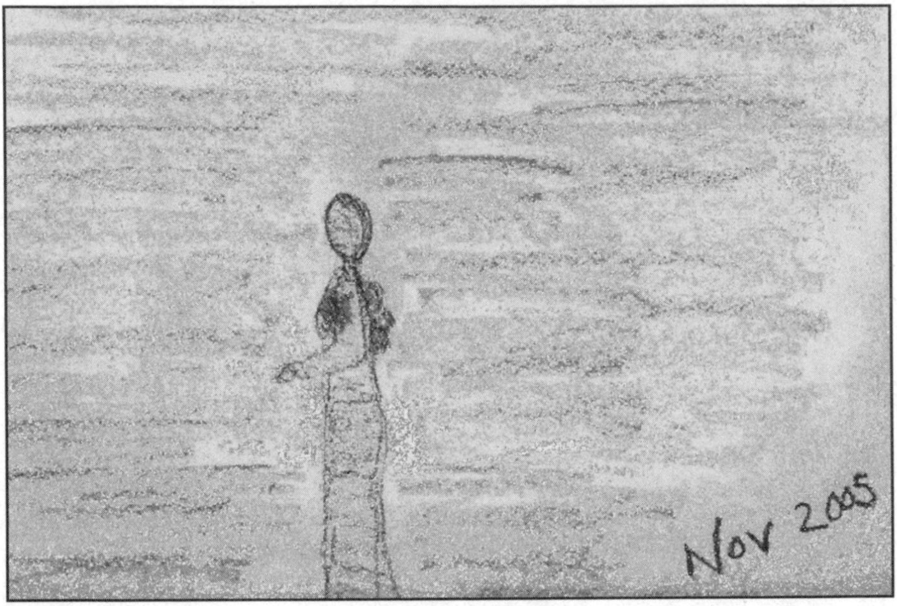

A Year in the Life of My Pain
Picture C

Picture C was made later in that year. It occurred to me that I'd never looked at what was inside my backpack! What was blocking me, I wondered. Fear. Fear was something that was always something external to me. In a meditation I decided to open the backpack, like a closet door. I opened it and was surprised to find nothing inside but dust. Why? Then I realized that my deepest pain was not physical, as I had originally thought—although I suffer severe physical pain— but emotional. My parents, but especially my mother, did not protect my heart. I realized my father was complicit in this situation also because he didn't know how to handle my mother and, to keep the peace, went along with what she was doing and agreed to stop showing love towards his daughters because that is what she requested saying, "It's not normal to hug and kiss your children and you must stop it." It broke my spirit, kept me down.

The realization that my emotional pain from my childhood was my deepest pain was such a light-bulb moment for me. Knowledge is power. I now had the knowledge of what was in my backpack. Wow! It was such a liberating moment. In Picture C, this is reflected in the light surrounding me and my backpack being smaller and now my heart isn't so dark. Only good can come of this knowledge. I can choose to make changes and look at the future with some optimism. I don't have all the answers yet but I have a starting point and that just feels so good.

It will be a long journey but one worth taking because I am certainly worth the effort. I have to give to myself what my parents did not give me. Stop playing the old tape recorder in my head and start a new one.

—Marie L., forty-three
Fibromyalgia Sufferer

And the insights Marie has garnered from her art still continue into the present. Months after rereading her statements above, Marie wrote us a note in which she described having "a new light-bulb moment." "I realized that that backpack wasn't just my backpack but it was my mother's backpack too, and my ancestors' backpack that I've been carrying all this time! Because they never dealt with their issues they passed it onto the next generation until someone says stop!!!! And I'm saying STOP!!! I'm not carrying your backpack and your garbage for you anymore! They are not mine to carry and I refuse to do it!! Wow! What a realization. The tough part is implementing that in my psyche every day but it's a start. Anyways, wow, this blows my mind!"

Cheryl

As mentioned earlier in chapter 7, Cheryl is one of the greatest success stories in our Mindfulness-Based Chronic Pain Management program. She went from being on disability, taking high doses of opioids, needing continuous oxygen due to her high opioid doses, and constant attendant care to reducing her medications by 90 percent, no longer needing oxygen, nor an attendant. After six years of living on disability income, she has recently returned to work. Interestingly, after doing our courses and reducing her medications, her head became clear enough to separate from, and then divorce, her unsupportive husband. This was when she made the most progress: when she was no longer enmeshed in what she describes as a "toxic relationship." Although her difficult marriage did not make her sick, it certainly played a huge role in keeping her in pain.

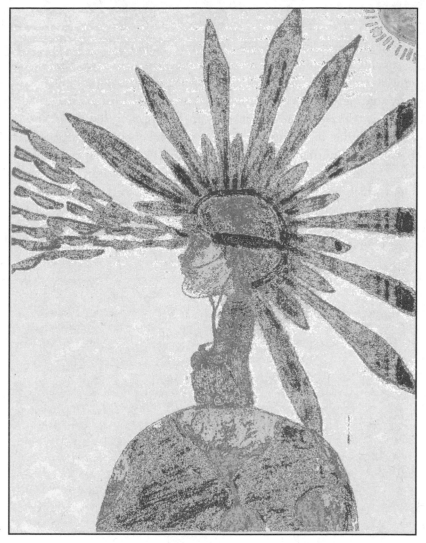

My Pain Experience

In my head there is a bandlike vise surrounding my head with daggers shooting into my eyes. Black shafts radiate from my head showing the intensity and severity of my pain. I'm standing on a globe that symbolizes being alone in the world or, at least, feeling like I am. My head is larger than the rest of my body (out of scale) to show the significance of where the pain is. Everything else is minute compared to my pain.

—Cheryl S., thirty-six
Severe Headaches Sufferer

Sharon

Sharon had had low-back pain ever since she injured herself lifting boxes while moving from one house to another. She was devastated that she could no longer perform her duties as a nurse in a neonatal unit. But her work, while rewarding, had been a constant reminder of the battles she'd had with miscarriages. She spent hours each day in bed, setting the alarm to get up just in time for her only daughter's return from school or her husband's return from work, not wanting them to know how much time she spent in bed. And she discovered more issues, buried deep in her subconscious, related to past traumas, which had likely led to her not healing from this physical pain.

My Bed

Sometimes I feel like a specimen in a jar. People observe me but can't help me. When I'm in my bed, I feel like I'm in a cocoon. Isolated. But after my meds and meditation I feel cozy and relaxed.

I'm Drowning in My Own Pain

Help! Help! Help! I'm drowning in my own pain. I'm Isolated and away from others.

> —Sharon K., forty-eight
> Back Pain Sufferer
> Now working with a therapist
> and making progress.

Lou

A large part of Lou's journey involved dealing with the emotional pain that had overshadowed her life; an emotional pain that had its roots as far back as her childhood. Crippled by arthritis in her knees and back, Lou was no longer able to escape her emotional challenges by extended travel, which had been her lifelong method for dealing with her emotional pain. A breast cancer survivor, she felt that if her emotional pain were not dealt with, she would have a relapse. *"The emotional pain is becoming larger whether I want it or not."*

When her mindfulness practice had made her aware of the extent of her depression, Lou decided to begin psychotherapy to learn new ways of dealing with her emotional pain. Today, Lou is a changed person. When she looked at an earlier picture she drew of her life, it brought her to tears realizing how far she's come in the two years since doing mindfulness training.

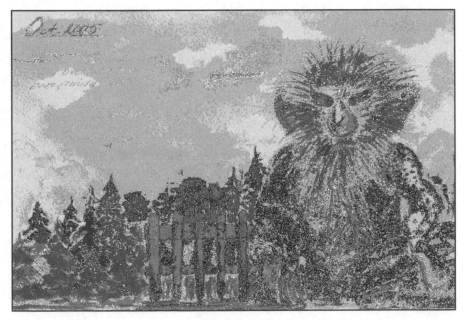

My Pain Troll

October 2005: My physical pain is ugly, always there, overrides everything else. Scary. It's like a troll. It's ugly and is with me at all times, but I can't get past him because he stands at my gate barring me from escaping toward living a joyful life and experiencing anything positive.

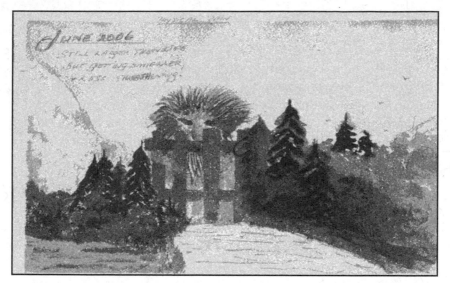

My Pain Troll

June 2006: My troll is getting smaller but he still fills my garden and makes it impossible for me to escape through the gate to other things.

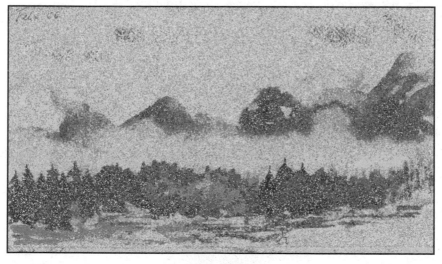

My Pain Troll

The troll is gone. I can see myself enjoying life—at last!
(See the small figure running at the bottom of the picture.)

—Lou O., seventy-five
Arthritis Sufferer

Al

Al started his pain journey after a motorcycle accident in his teens when he damaged his back and was unable to walk properly for some months. Although he recovered completely, he started getting severe back pain again when he hurt his back clearing ice from his driveway at age forty. He later had surgery that performed a back fusion, but pain has persisted in his lower back and neck.

I have a background in drafting and engineering for a manufacturing company, and creating charts and graphs comes naturally to me. I had no idea what to draw until I flipped through my day timer and noticed that I wrote my pain scores from zero to ten each day. I then charted my pain scores over a thirty-day period onto a graph. Then, playing with the graphic, I noticed that there is a center to my being that looks like a spine and it goes up the middle of the page. I thought about the days when my pain is high, and realized that I withdraw from the world on those days. The more pain I'm in, the more pain medication I take, and the more I withdraw. I don't talk to my family, I remain solemn, I'm surly with my wife (which isn't good), and I generally hold all the people I love and everything else in the world I enjoy, away from me.

—Al R., fifty-three
Degenerating Joint Disease
(Unexplained)

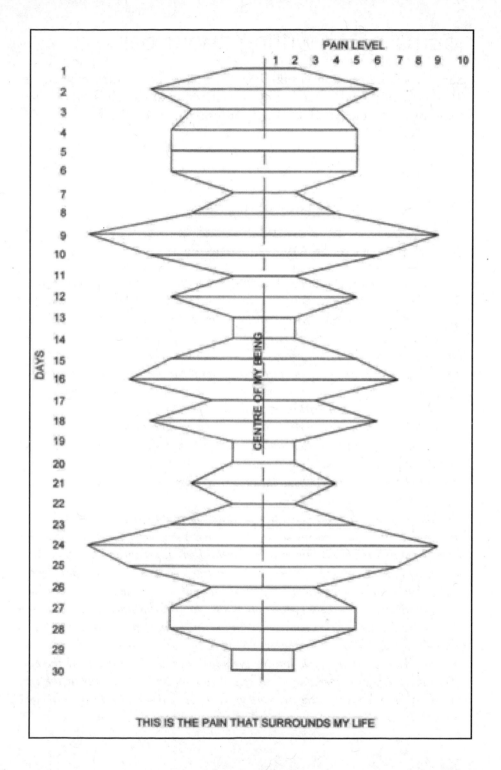

PAIN LEVEL

THIS IS THE PAIN THAT SURROUNDS MY LIFE

journaling or writing about pain

Some people are never able to think in pictures or draw pictures of any type. They may, on the other hand, do very well with writing. Chris, who suffers from migraines, preferred to write about his pain.

Chris

Chris is a severe migraine sufferer.

A Verbal Picture of My Migraine Pain

I am standing in a white space; no visible light source, simply stark white light as far as the eye can see in all directions; so bright as to be painful, and without the relief of being able to close my eyelids for even the shortest of moments. The only thing in existence, other than myself, is a group of people off in the distance, so far away that no individual person can be discerned. They are all surrounded by a thick fog that occasionally completely obscures them from view but, more often than not, they are there. I know only instinctively that this group is made up of friends (what few I have left), family (from as far away as Europe; even those of whom I have only heard stories... but all, I know, are aware of my situation), and my doctors. I can tell that they are intensely sad and frustrated at the fact that they are all, somehow, being held back from getting any closer and providing comfort and aid, no matter how hard they try. They weep but never cease trying to reach me.

The physical pain manifests itself in the form of an old-style leather football helmet. It is two sizes too small for me but has somehow been made to fit my head. Now that it's on, it cannot be removed. There is a visor on the helmet that covers my eyes. There are vise-like screws in front of each eye, and they tighten and loosen at their own will in an attempt to push my eyeballs to the very back of my head and crush them against my skull. None of this affects my vision and the light continues to shine painfully. Within this helmet, there are a number of one-inch-wide and one-inch-long, razor-sharp steel spikes that embed themselves into my head; at each temple, on the eyebrow ridge above each eye, at the base of my skull; one on either side of my spinal column and a final one at the very top of my head for good measure. No blood, simply pain, and no way to remove the helmet.

Attached to the helmet is a heavy, thick wrought-iron chain and somehow I am prevented from lowering myself to the floor to lighten the load. The chain, in turn, is attached to a great weight, the style of which you might see in a Bugs Bunny cartoon. This then prevents me from accessing the group in the distance, or even seeking out relief from the light. Floating in front of me, within easy reach, is a veritable pharmacopoeia. I know that it holds every type of treatment and medication used to treat my condition, and then some. I'm also aware of the fact that the best result I can hope for from any combination thereof would be that the size of the helmet would increase to being only one size too small and, perhaps, one or two of its spikes might recede slightly, all for a matter of, perhaps, two or three hours.

Also available are the drugs that, again, only for a matter of hours, will allow me to be free of the anchoring chair, and allow me to ignore the pain somewhat and function, to some small degree, amongst the distant crowd even though the fog is thicker, even as the brightness never really recedes. The evils of these medications can easily outweigh any benefits I receive from them unless constantly monitored and metered. This is my pain.

—Chris R., thirty-six
Migraine Sufferer

Denise

Ironically, Denise always used to look down on people with disabilities, always believing that if they could just "get a grip," they could function in life and not have to depend on others. Then nine months ago, Denise, now in her fifties, suddenly came down with a bad case of "flu." When the flu and exhaustion didn't pass, she was diagnosed with chronic fatigue syndrome (CFS). Her doctor said there really wasn't much she could do other than rest, and referred her to our mindfulness program. She dragged herself to the first class uncertain that anything would come of it and started reading Jon Kabat-Zinn's book, *Full Catastrophe Living*. "All of a sudden" she says, she had a "realization" that she had been beating herself up her entire life. When she encountered any problems in life, she would "solve it by working harder." Then she became ill and for the first time she realized if she worked harder, she would become "more ill."

Being a teacher of adult literacy, it came naturally for Denise to write a poem about her experience. It arose spontaneously while she was musing about her pain and the stresses in life. She began to imagine her pain as a terrorist whose chief weapon is fear. The only way to disarm a terrorist, she thought, was to no longer generate fear. It was at that moment that Denise began the challenging work of disarming herself from the fear she had carried along her entire life. And then the poem, she says, "just clicked."

My Pain

My pain is a terrorist
choosing strategic targets
hurting me
using guerilla tactics
entirely without conscience
an alien force, moving in stealth
hitting here, hitting there
causing me fear.

My pain represents the catastrophic axis of evil
And my hypothalamic-pituitary-adrenal axis
lives in fear, in terror
it attacks, then flees
attacks again, a mercenary
working for pathogenic stress incorporated
entirely without conscience
it thrives on my fear, my reactions
it uses heinous weapons.

My weapons fail
drugs cause collateral damage
my immunity is confused
intelligence is compromised
pain prevails
entirely without conscience
yet there is no surrender.

A new weapon
a powerful mindful resistance
nothing to fear but fear itself
peace on my terms
acknowledging the pain

giving it a place in my world
but taking away its weapons, accepting its gifts,
understanding that it does have a conscience
détente, a truce, peace.

—Denise T., fifty
Chronic Fatigue and Fibromyalgia
Sufferer

A month ago Denise went to a fibromyalgia specialist who told her she was recovering exceptionally well and could expect to return to work within a year. Denise now feels that her illness has been a gift in a number of ways, because deep down she was not a "compassionate" person when it came to other people. The imposition on her physical activities by the CFS has caused her to look at the world through a very different lens now. "It is gift because it can help me from damaging myself further over time. I still get quite tired but now I listen to my body and tell myself I must listen to it and lie down and rest."

For the most part, Denise no longer needs pain medications to control her pain. "I used to be taking handsful," she admits. She's returning her attention to the house she and her partner are building in the country and plan to retire to in a few years. She gives herself permission to not have to work "sixteen hours a day on the house while it is under construction," and to rest when she needs to. "It will get done when it gets done. My whole life has been a race. In fact, I ran ten marathons. They were pretty much a metaphor with what I was doing to myself generally."

Denise now realizes that as a result of a very difficult childhood, she learned to compensate for her difficult life by her overactivity. She was keeping busy to escape the "terrorists of her past." She now realizes that the psychological pain of her childhood was probably bigger, in the final analysis, than her CFS pain and that it probably led to her getting CFS. Her mindful practices now help her deal with her psychological pain and now, whenever she thinks about the past, she no longer blames herself or beats herself up. "I forget that it's gone, it's past, and there's no point in fussing about it. It's gone."

Expressing Your Pain or Mood on Paper

There are many benefits to be gained by expressing yourself creatively through artwork or writing. Some of those benefits are briefly described below.

Pain awareness and stress. Many people say that they experience less pain when absorbed in an activity—any activity—including art. When done mindfully, making art can reduce stress, and in some cases, completely eliminate the awareness of pain.

Mood. You might also use art to express your usual mood. Artwork can depict your usual mood state, which might be a mood that everyone else is aware of, except you yourself. By seeing that, you might be able to change your mood and break the cycle of your suffering by finding alternate ways of dealing with the difficult parts of your life.

Reaching out. Making art can become a powerful way of connecting you to other people and it can help them understand what you are experiencing. Your artwork can give other people in your life a way of helping you decode the various levels of meaning in your creation.

Helping others. Making art can also help others in chronic pain relate to and benefit from seeing your creativity about your own pain, and your artwork may inspire them to become creative too, and thus derive their own benefits from creativity.

Now It's Your Turn

It's time now to do some of your own artwork, either on paper, as a model, a collage, a poem or whatever feels right to you. Don't worry if it doesn't come through straight away; do it when you're ready. And hold onto what you create. Then a few months after you finish it, go back and do another, and then another. You'll be illustrating or chronicling your own journey, and you may find that you understand yourself and your situation very much better by doing this.

Making art can become an important way to become aware of your progress over time. Many pain sufferers do not have an objective way of measuring their progress. Engaging in artistic expression can show you how you are progressing with your pain management.

Therapists have worked with children in this way for years. Perhaps it's the children's wonderful beginner's mind that allows them to express themselves so freely and truthfully in this manner, but it can certainly work for adults too, especially now that you are cultivating beginner's mind. Making art is a powerful way to help you arrive at something our pain patients tell us is very difficult, but very necessary; that is, acceptance.

Acceptance Through Art

Acceptance means quite simply accepting things the way they are in this moment, while realizing it's not necessarily how they are going to be forever. Ironically, it seems that arriving at acceptance is the gateway to moving forward. Your artwork will help you to see the way things are right now, and it may open up new ideas about moving forward for you. Or it may help you to find closure for some of your disappointments. Your artwork can also provide you with a way to grieve for the way things were—a bereavement.

Perhaps you might take some time to continue your mindfulness practice and to get your artwork done before you move onto the final chapters. Do some visualizations or imagery of your pain and then reframe your physical pain as part of your life. Remember, there's no rush. Life is here for the reclaiming, either with chronic pain or with less of it.

Chapter 11

visualizations and guided imagery

To accomplish great things we must first dream, then visualize, then plan, believe, act.

—Alfred A. Montapert

Imagery has been considered an important healing tool in virtually all of the world's cultures. Navajo Indians, for example, practice an elaborate form of imagery that encourages a person to "see" her or himself as healthy. Ancient Egyptians and Greeks, including Aristotle and Hippocrates, believed that visualizing disease caused the body to experience illness and pain whereas visualizing health restored the body to wellness. As a chronic pain sufferer, you may be open to learning how you too can use this powerful tool to deal more effectively with your pain. Visualization and guided imagery are often used as interchangeable terms, but in our practice we use them in slightly different contexts.

Imagining your body and mind structures so that you can then alter them in a positive way, such as boosting your immune system, is what we call *guided imagery*. In the immune system, *natural killer cells* (NK cells) are an important component because they can recognize and destroy virus-infected cells and other invaders. Danish researchers Zachariae and colleagues (1990) found increased natural killer cell activity in ten college students who'd been asked to imagine their immune systems were becoming very effective.

Another study in the U.S., by Andrews and Hall (1990) found that people who suffered from recurrent canker sores in their mouths significantly reduced the frequency of their outbreaks after they began visualizing their sores being bathed in a soothing coating of white cells. And at the University of South Florida, Moody, Fraser, and Yarandi (1993) reported that nineteen individuals with bronchitis and emphysema significantly improved the quality of their lives, eased their pain, and lifted their depression by using guided imagery.

Visualization is the term we use to describe imagining being somewhere or with someone either playing out a scenario or just experiencing the scene. The usual pleasant mood and improved emotional state that may be associated with such a scenario tend to be experienced during a visualization. When you're in a positive emotional state, generally, you feel better and may have less pain, and your mood enhances the functioning of all of your body systems.

mindfulness, guided imagery, and visualization: do they fit together?

Mindfulness is being fully present in the present moment with whatever comes up, good or bad—wherever you are. So some people question whether visualizations and guided imagery are *anti*mindfulness practices. We say they are philosophically compatible. You start with what *is,* and using the power of your mind you first focus on the way it is now. You note the changes in each moment as you experience each moment, and you take the changes in a positive direction, noting the negative emotions associated with the unpleasant sensation of pain.

These techniques have been around for a long time and perhaps are best known for their use in cancer studies, but we didn't start using guided imagery until about a year into our mindfulness courses with our patients. Michael was the first patient to try it in one of our classes.

Michael

As we were finishing a meditation and heading into our discussion period in class, we felt there was more pain in the room than usual. Michael was about to have one of his painful spasm attacks that look like seizures but are really a form of pseudoseizure involving electric shocks coursing through his body, lasting up to twenty minutes at a time. These attacks had limited his life terribly because he never knew when one would occur. He could be caught by an attack on the street, in a taxi, at a movie, just about anywhere. When we looked around the room and saw the tense faces of others in pain too, we made a quick change of plan.

We told them to close their eyes again and, for the first time, we gently talked them through visualizing their pain as something tangible they were familiar with—some object that they could compare to their pain, such as fire or ice, or a stabbing knife. And then they were to look head-on at the object representing their pain, whatever and wherever it was, and imagine it evaporating or stopping, and taking away their fear and dread. After five to ten minutes we opened our eyes; the faces in the classroom were more relaxed, and Michael was okay. He had imagined an electrical circuit board malfunctioning and sparking, and in his mind's eye, he had used an electrical fire extinguisher to stop it—and his pain was subsiding. Several others reported similar results.

The next day at home it took him twenty minutes to do what we had done with the class in ten minutes, but Michael was on a roll. Two days later, in Saturday's maintenance meditation class, he started another attack. We knelt beside him as others around us did a walking meditation, and we slowly talked him through the imagery again. The attack subsided.

At the next class, we encountered him outside beaming. He was getting great results with practice. He recounted how he'd had a pending attack at the same time a migraine was beginning, a few days earlier. He had again visualized using a fire extinguisher for electrical fires on his attack. Then he'd turned his attention to his migraine. He'd imagined it as a fire, and in his mind's eye, he took a blanket, soaked it in water, and used it to smother the fire. In fifteen minutes his migraine was gone! He'd experienced having power over his pain for the first time in his life!

Michael went on to become skillful at helping others with suggestions on how they could picture their pain and imagine an antidote to counteract it. One of our favorites was imagining pain as an hourglass or egg timer, and watching the pain diminish as the sand flowed into the bottom of the hourglass.

The artwork you've made may help you with finding images that best fit your pain. Your focus can start with your breath, as in your other meditations, but move on to focus on the image you create of your pain. This process works just as well for emotional pain as it does for physical pain. For example, for emotional pain, you might imagine a tangled ball of black knitting yarn sitting in your brain, where you identify one end of it and gradually unravel it to fashion into a tidy properly wound ball instead.

The following meditation is an example of guided imagery you can try for your pain. Most people find that a twenty-to-thirty-minute guided imagery meditation is the most helpful. But by slowing down your thoughts it can be done over a longer period of time, if that is what you want to do. You can find five- and fifteen-minute guided imagery meditations for pain on the CD: *Pain Speaking*, CD number 4. The information you need to purchase the CD can be found in the Recommended Reading section in the back of this book.

Guided Imagery Meditation

This is a guided imagery
For emotional or physical pain.
So find a quiet place, if one is available
And if not, just create one inside of yourself.

Get into a position that allows you the most comfort
At this time.
Make sure you're not disturbed
And then
When you are ready
Just go to your breath
And observe it.
Whether at the level of the nostrils
Or the mouth
Or the chest
Or the abdomen
Wherever it feels comfortable for you.

Perhaps work on slowing your breath down
If it seems too fast.
Ground yourself in the present moment.
Not trying to get anywhere fast
Just being patient
Committed.

Breathing in
And breathing out.

And when you are ready
Take your mind's eye over
To where the pain is.
Bringing awareness to it.
Observing it.
Imagining walking around it
And seeing it from every angle.

Not afraid
Not dreading its potential and the emotions associated with it.
Not giving it power.

Just look at it
As if you were seeing it for the first time
With beginner's mind.
Breathing.

Becoming aware of what the sensation of pain is like for you
Without emotions amplifying it.

Perhaps it is aching
Like a bad toothache.

Or sore and inflamed
As in a swollen reddened joint.

Perhaps it is twisting
Like a hand twisting a towel

Tighter and tighter.
Or stabbing like a knife.

Perhaps it is burning
Like a fire.

Or scalding like boiling water.

Or perhaps it feels like electric shocks
On a malfunctioning circuit board.

Perhaps your pain is like a jagged block of ice.
Perhaps it is tight and spasming
As if it were being stretched
Like a rubber band.

Or perhaps you feel as though you are being
Sliced or cut.
Perhaps your pain is throbbing
Keeping pace with your beating heart.
Whatever it feels like
It is time to take an image
That best fits your pain
And in your mind's eye
Work with it
To undo, unwind, what is being done.

Perhaps you might imagine
Gently rubbing a soothing balm
Into the aching part of you
Dissolving the pain as it absorbs
Into your skin.

Perhaps you place an ice pack
On your inflamed joint.

Perhaps a gentle hand grasps the hand
That is twisting the painful part of you
And stops its action.

Or stays the hand
That holds the knife.

Perhaps you can imagine
Soaking a blanket in water
And throwing it over the fire of your pain.

Perhaps you find an extinguisher for electrical fires
And spray it over your electric-shocklike pains
Until they die down.

Perhaps your jagged block of ice
Melts
As you breathe warmth over it.

Perhaps you can imagine
Massaging soothing creams into tight muscles
And feeling them gradually
Little by little
Relax.

Aware of whatever feels right for your pain.
Taking a few minutes now
In silence
To work with its undoing.

SILENCE

Dissolving

Fragmenting

Disintegrating

Melting

Softening

Undoing

Fading

Untwisting

Drifting away

The color red changing to blue and green

Pain diminishing, receding

Shrinking in front of your gaze

Aware of not feeling threatened by the pain
Not fearing it
Not recoiling from it
Just being with it
As it dies down
Perhaps like a piece of discordant music
Difficult to listen to
Fading into silence.
The silence of peace.
The silence of safety.

Some people take to guided imagery faster than others and we've wondered if that is because some individuals think naturally in pictures, while others think naturally in words. However, some who found guided imagery hard to do at first, have reported that it gets easier with practice and they can indeed do it.

Belleruth Naperstek, a psychotherapist and pioneer in guided imagery, has written more extensively on this subject in *Staying Well with Guided Imagery: How to Harness the Power of Your Imagination for Health and Healing* (1994). You might want to use her book to get more help with imagining the parts of your body that you need to heal.

visualization

In our work we use the term "visualization" to describe two of the most popular meditations Jon Kabat-Zinn narrated over a twenty-minute period: a lake meditation and a mountain meditation. We composed and added another called the room meditation.

In each case, some of the power derived from these meditations is similar to the benefit you derive from listening to music you like: that is, the power to be inspired and change your mood to a more positive one. Your body-mind functions so much better when you feel good, and as a result you cope with pain better.

The Lake Meditation

This wonderful meditation, traditionally done lying down, involves building a picture in your mind's eye of a lake, which you may have seen or perhaps imagined. Lake scenes are commonly associated with peace and a feeling of contentment, but if you have had a bad experience at a lake or with water, this might not be the best meditation option for you. We say this because some of our patients have not taken well to this meditation when they've had previously bad associations with water. As an alternative, you might sit on the bank and contemplate your lake when you start to practice this meditation and, later on, you might feel more comfortable with "becoming" the lake.

You may have wonderful childhood memories of going to a summer cottage on a lake with your family. The power of your thoughts can be so great that you might observe that even thinking about the good times you had back then, puts you in a better mood and causes you to feel more relaxed. That's a good start: you cope better with pain when you are relaxed. But seeing the analogy between the lake and your body and mind is what is really being sought here.

In this visualization, you imagine the "weather" of your life as happening above the surface of your lake (which is you). The weather whips the surface of the lake to form waves and frothing waters, while in the deeper recesses of the lake only gentle undulations take place. The idea is that with consistent mindfulness practice, when challenges do occur in your life—as they inevitably will—you become like the deeper recesses of your lake, with only gentle undulations of your body and mind systems responding to the stressors around you. This is a much healthier way to respond to stress. But it takes practice.

The Mountain Meditation

The mountain meditation is another one of Jon Kabat-Zinn's meditations. This one is done in a sitting position, if possible. You sit cross-legged on the floor, and visualize yourself as a mountain, with all of a mountain's strength and beauty. Your head is the peak of the mountain, and your bottom is the mountain's base. Once again, the weather—which changes all the time around your mountain—is the analogy with the stressors and challenges of your life; the seasons are analogous to your changing life circumstances, and you become the mountain, with the strength to stay grounded despite all the wild weather patterns that may be going on around you.

Some people find that this meditation empowers them. Doing it makes them feel less helpless against their pain challenges, which are now readily linked with emotional life events when exacerbations of pain occur. But as with the lake meditation, there are some who have an adverse reaction to practicing this meditation if, for example, they were always called on to be the strong one in their family or circle friends, and never allowed to show any weaknesses. That awareness brings insight.

The Room Meditation

This meditation is designed to allow you to meet with your core "self." It is best done after you have been meditating for a while because there may be some emotional discomfort if you try doing this meditation too early in your mindfulness practice. It can be done in whatever position you find comfortable, providing you are in a dignified posture that allows the unrestricted flow of blood throughout your body.

First, you are encouraged to design a personal space that might be a room or a small walled garden. Or you might design a personal space in a boat anchored in the middle of a lake. Or you might design a cottage in a field or a forest. You go on to design the entrance to your space, and to decide the colors and textures of everything; the walls, ceiling, windows, and furnishings. You even to decide whether you will have refreshments in there—or paper, pens, and drawing materials. While you are focusing on the details of your room, the weather of your life is going on outside the room leaving you, for the moment, free to focus on the "now."

After all the details of your personal space have been settled, you then decide whether you will sit or stand for your meeting with your "self." And then, you imagine a "shimmering" taking place as your "self" separates from you, and you are standing in front of your self, looking into your own eyes nonjudgmentally.

Then it is time to communicate; through speaking, drawing, writing to each other, or touching. You may continue communicating for several minutes in silence. You may see your core self as looking the way you appear now, or as you looked when you were a child. Sometimes, seeing yourself as a child takes your "self" back to the time before some of your most intense life challenges occurred. It's sort of like seeing what you were like before you were "wounded." If this does happen to you, you take advantage of the fact that you are now an adult: older, wiser, and with more emotional resources. You might take that young "you" by the hand and offer the nurturing you needed so badly at that vulnerable age, and did not receive.

As the meeting with your core self comes to an end, you take your leave. The shimmering takes place again as "self" merges with who you are. You turn toward your exit and slowly walk in that direction, preparing to reenter the world. Every action observed, every step takes you out toward the challenges—the "weather" of your life.

You will likely find this to be a profound meditation but, again, it takes practice. If you turned this visualization into an unpleasant experience, this is a great moment to ask yourself, "Why?" Did you not deserve to have a good experience when you had all those choices to make so freely? What was that about? The room meditation is available from www.painspeaking.com.

If it was a helpful experience and you enjoyed being in your space, you might choose to return to it for many brief visits now that you've designed and built it. Of course, there are those who redesign their spaces, and it may change from year to year, or even from month to month. Always be curious: Why have you changed it? What have you learned by asking that question? If you find this meditation quite traumatic, ensure that you discuss your feelings with your physician or therapist. But understand that even if it created very difficult feelings, it is probably important to the future quality of your life that you patiently "sit" with them, when you feel able, to allow yourself to move forward. Your very awareness is important, but like dipping your toe in the water to test the temperature before you plunge in, you can do that here too.

As Socrates famously said, "The unexamined life is not worth living."

next steps

In the next and final chapter you can see how you are doing with your mindfulness practice, and assess the impact it has had on your pain and suffering so far. We will also comment on some of the medication interventions you might need to help you cross the bridge from suffering pain, to living more comfortably with pain, or to living with less pain. We've helped you to harness your inner resources so that you will depend less on the external ones. You're in the home stretch: On a course to find balance in your life; the balance that has been missing through lack of awareness and which is now there for the taking—with pain or without it.

Chapter 12

reclaiming your life:
with pain or without

Not everything that is faced can be changed, but nothing
can be changed until it is faced.

—James Baldwin

Has your relationship with your pain changed since you began reading and
working with this book? If you truly committed to doing the work of cultivating your own mindfulness practice while learning why you should do this
work, we're betting it has. And by now, most likely you understand that as
your mood and emotions change from moment to moment—so do your body
systems—including your immune system, which fluctuates in its efficiency
and effectiveness depending on your stress levels.

Your ability to heal, fight infection, and protect yourself from cancers and
other illnesses is likely intimately associated with how much emotional and
physical pain you feel. Moreover, your health and pain conditions are greatly
influenced by the emotional stress you feel when encountering your day-to-
day challenges as well as your physical stressors, such as the quality of your
nutrition and sleep, and your ability to move.

Furthermore, it's likely that you become even more sensitive to stress
as one stressor builds on another, causing you to become more and more

susceptible. Your susceptibility leads to less sleep, less tolerance for other stressors, and a poorer functioning immune system. Like falling dominoes, these lead to less exercise, weaker muscles, and less tolerance for activity. Then you have fewer outings, less interpersonal contact, and fewer interactions with others. The result of all of this is more sadness, greater likelihood of depression, and on and on and on. Soon your disability is mainly composed of your losses, which all occurred after your initial injury or illness.

We think that the chief reason some people choose not to continue in our program beyond their first three or four classes, is likely that they are not ready to do the work, not ready to invest the time, and surprisingly for some, not ready to give up their pain. Yes, we have actually seen people having meltdowns when they were asked to imagine life without their pain. And when you think about it carefully, it's not that hard to understand.

subconscious "secondary gain"

Secondary gain is the term used by health care professionals and others to describe the state of staying sick in order to continue on disability, and to avoid having to act, live, behave, and work like a fully able person. Consequently, it's often used as a derogatory term. Suppose you've suffered from pain for ten years and haven't been in the workforce for eight. You have a constant disability income coming in, not that much, but you've downsized your life to cope.

You go to bed later than most, rise later than most, and others in your life have accommodated to the fact that you need some help and concessions. It takes you much longer to accomplish tasks that you remember you used to do very quickly. You know the job you used to do has evolved into something very different since the technology explosion. So if you woke up tomorrow with no pain, and you got a phone call or an e-mail telling you to report for work on Monday, you'd likely feel pretty anxious. Your pain just might come back, especially if you subconsciously go looking for it in desperation. All of a sudden, your pain has become your friend, not your foe. It legitimizes you being on disability. After all, you still think a blackberry is a fruit!

You've met Michael before in this book. He was with us as a patient in the early days of our mindfulness program. He was the patient described in chapter 11 who visualized a circuit board malfunctioning and used an imaginary electrical fire extinguisher to stop the malfunction. By doing this, he learned how to control his pain with guided imagery. He has been both an inspiration and a lesson to us in the art of "letting go." Ultimately, however, we could not "rescue" him from his pain.

Michael

Michael had been seeking help for many years when he was first seen at our pain clinic. He had not worked in fourteen years because of the pain in many areas of his body. He also suffered attacks that appeared to be seizures, which came on suddenly as painful spasms coursed through his body for as long as ten to twenty minutes at a time. His sister had been diagnosed with multiple sclerosis (MS) and his symptoms were similar, but his tests in the past had not confirmed this.

So he belonged to no particular specialty, and was in that frustrating place of being in pain without a diagnosis to make the pain respectable. In fact, he felt scorned by neurologists and knew that many health care professionals thought he was fabricating the attacks he suffered. But even with no diagnosis, his pain still had to be managed.

We worked with the pain medications to find the best ones for him and at the same time he signed up for our classes in mindfulness. Over the next two years we saw a transformation take place as Michael learned how to control his pain through mindfulness.

He had stopped working due to increasing bodily pain only a few months after his marriage fifteen years earlier, and had not been able to work full-time for the last fourteen years. Stress at home had also played a part. His wife hated her job and suffered from headaches and depression. He felt responsible for her being trapped in a job with a boss she disliked, but she was too depressed to look for anything else. And, in truth, she did resent having to head out to work every day leaving her husband engrossed in The Price Is Right *on TV.*

During his meditation courses he also became aware that he had big issues with his father over matters that had happened between them in the past, and over time he managed to forgive his father and to reconcile. That helped his state of mind a lot.

We sometimes introduced new ideas in class. One day we asked the participants to imagine for two minutes what they would do with their lives if they awoke one morning without pain. Although some enjoyed the exercise, three participants, including Michael, had virtual panic attacks. He realized his whole life was structured around his illness. He believed that after all this time he had no skills to reenter the workforce. It took him several weeks to get over this revelation. He felt useless and he spoke of his low regard for himself.

A few months later, he had two weeks free from pain for the first time in fifteen years, but then it returned as intensely as before. However, Michael said that his relationship with his pain had changed: he was not as afraid of it anymore. And then he discovered the power of the guided imagery described in chapter 11. His attacks subsided. For the first time in his life he began to feel that he had power over his pain.

For a few months he became 90 percent pain-free, on a fraction of the medication he had been on two years earlier. He had the body language of a much more self-confident person. But when he started to consider going back into the workforce, he became anxious and depressed again.

How would he manage after so many years away from the discipline of work? So much had changed. Like others who have been on disability for a long time, he was very afraid of not finding a job and very afraid of failure. He tried sending out résumés again: good ones, which his wife helped him to compose. But there were no phone calls.

Feeling defeated, his need for pain medications rose again. One year later his wife chose to separate. They have been apart for two years now, and he lives in a rooming house with others who have mental and other health challenges. Pain is ever-present. He feels that he has given up the quest for better health.

Michael's case illustrates the phenomenon of completely unconscious secondary gain. And perhaps this is where the medical profession and rehabilitation institutions fall short: perhaps we needed to take him out there and get him a job, convincing a prospective employer to hire him for a month without pay, until he was able to demonstrate that he could do it. It's likely that everyone going through a rehabilitation program should be introduced to work straight away, not left to deteriorate for the few months or weeks intervening between receiving the rehabilitation services and finding a job. It's just too likely that returning to the absence of routine, reduced strength, and motivation will bring back the pain at the intense levels that initially crafted the disability, which followed the injury, accident or illness.

visiting the doctor: you and your emotions

After being in pain for as long as you have, you also may not be aware that you have exhibited certain behaviors that aren't helping you get the help you need. For example, anger is frequently an emotion patients bring in with them to a clinic and, however subliminal and unaware of it you may be, anger can be repellent to health care professionals—who may not have identified it specifically—except to know they feel uncomfortable around you.

Our colleagues intuitively know that you are less likely to benefit from certain procedures, such as nerve blocks, if you are going through too much psychological distress, and you may not be offered a procedure that might have been offered if your anger had not been sensed. This may not seem fair, but the reality is there is a reduced likelihood of achieving better pain management in the presence of anger (Sarno 1998). Additionally, we find it draining and futile to try to treat angry patients with pain medications, which don't work as well in the presence of anger, without helping them to notice and deal with their anger as well. Your anger may be harming your chances of finding work too.

Sandra

Sandra was very hard to convince to take the mindfulness classes—she'd been in counseling for many years, she said, and really didn't need any more psychological interventions. She was a severe migraine sufferer, who had worked full-time most of the time we knew her. She was on very large doses of pain medication, although not visiting the ER on as regular a basis as she had been before she became our patient.

But one day she came in very distressed: she had been laid off from her second job in the past three years. Warning bells went off in our heads. She had been in quite a high-level position in a large company, and we'd thought that the first layoff was due to downsizing. She'd managed to find a second job just before her benefits were cut off from the first job, which was a huge relief because her drug bills were so high.

But now, a year later, she received another layoff notice. What was happening? She hadn't missed much time from work as she was stoic and had worked through her migraines as best she'd been able, using her medications to reduce her pain. We advised a tearful Sandra, "Start our mindfulness classes—we're just about to start a new course now." She couldn't argue now that she didn't have the time.

Her body language was rather stiff, perhaps resistant and somewhat angry, during the first and second classes but she did her meditations daily. And by the third class, she was amusing us by bringing in her floor cleaner to clean the floor before class started. She didn't consider the room clean enough for class members to lay their mats on the floor for meditation practice after the medical residents had their lunch rounds there earlier in the day. Toward the end of classes her body language had become noticeably different. In her next consultation, Sandra acknowledged that she had been able to tap into some really important feelings through meditation—for example, real anger toward her mother. She'd always known she'd had problems with how critical her mother had been of her, and she'd thought that she'd dealt with them in the past with therapy.

However, in her meditations she'd seen that some of her anger was nonverbal—it was still an issue. Sensibly, she had turned to counseling again to augment her meditation practice, and was now feeling happier. Her migraines became less aggressive. She had more control over them. She also came to realize that her bottled-up anger had probably played a role in her relationships with her bosses at work, and may have led to her layoffs.

The following Christmas, when her adult son visited, she waited a few days before asking him if he'd noticed anything different about her. Awkwardly he said he had—she seemed less angry. "So why didn't you say something earlier?" she asked. "I thought you'd be angry," he replied sheepishly!

Over the next few years, Sandra encountered some major challenges including bankruptcy, eviction from her apartment, and the possible recurrence of an old lung cancer lesion seen on a chest X-ray. But she used her meditation practice to meet each event with courage, and she got through successfully. Perhaps losing that second job actually helped her to change her life.

Helplessness and Hopelessness

Two other adverse emotions we often see, which are correlated with a poor outcome, are helplessness and hopelessness. After years of not being able to recover to your pre-accident or pre-illness state, helplessness is very understandable; however, it is an immensely adverse emotion capable of doing a lot of sabotage to your body's ability to heal.

Martin Seligman, a renowned psychologist, described his interesting research in *Learned Optimism* (1990). He devised a model to study helplessness using three groups of dogs. One group was shocked with an electric current; but the dogs learned to stop the shock by pushing a panel with their noses that stopped the current. Another group was shocked but they could do nothing about stopping the shocks, and a control group got no shocks all.

When the dogs that had learned to control the shocks with their noses were put into a box with a partition, across which they could climb to escape further shocks, they easily climbed across the partition to the no-shock or safe side. The control group also climbed over the partition easily when they were shocked. But most of the dogs that had had no control in the first part of the experiment never found the "safe" side of the box. They just lay down and gave up.

Seligman found, however, that by repeating the experiment and physically carrying the helpless group back and forth over the partition to demonstrate the safe side, the dogs, which had formerly given up, learned how to climb over the partition. They learned to reverse their helpless response. Furthermore, Seligman found that puppies that were taught to respond actively appeared to be immunized against learned helplessness as adults.

These experiments were extended in a different form to humans by Donald Hiroto who was Seligman's colleague (Seligman 1990). He worked with human volunteers by exposing them to loud noises. One group learned to stop the noise. Another had no control over the noise at all. The third group, the controls, were not exposed to loud noise. Then the three groups were given a partitioned shuttle box: if they put their hand on one side, they could cause an annoying wooshing sound. By changing their hand to the other side, they could make the noise stop.

As in the dog experiment, the majority of the group that originally lacked any control over the loud noise just left their hand on the side with the annoying sound, and didn't even try to move it. The two other groups moved their hands quickly to the other side. In both the human and the dog experiments, about one in three of those in the "helpless" group did not become helpless and found their way to deal with the stressor. These results were repeated in other experiments. Moreover, in the control groups of both dogs and humans where neither shocks nor loud noises were administered, about one in ten, exhibited "helpless" behavior and did not move.

It's likely that this behavior reflects what may occur in both the general population and our population of pain sufferers. Some instinctively learn how to "change" their minds; that is, how to take "baby steps," which become steadier and stronger, and eventually lead to a more normal and productive life. Others may never take those steps, but we wonder whether they might, if they were provided with enthusiastic life coaches to "lift them over the partition." And perhaps mindfulness helps people to become aware that the partition exists and can be crossed.

Seligman's thesis is that becoming resilient to stress, even optimistic, is a skill that can be taught, paving the way for programs like our Mindfulness-Based Chronic Pain Management classes.

Helplessness, the magnification of pain, and ruminations about pain are all measured on a scale devised by Michael Sullivan and coworkers (1995) called the Pain Catastrophizing Scale. Using this scale, our research has shown these unhelpful thought processes are reduced a lot, statistically and significantly, by going through our Mindfulness-Based Chronic Pain Management course.

One sad couple who came to our chronic pain management classes, driving two hours to get there each week, entered the first week looking both helpless and hopeless. Melinda had been in pain since an accident in the 1980s and her husband was attending class to support her, as well as drive her to the course. Halfway through the course when we had the class doing artwork to express their pain, she wrote her own epitaph instead of depicting her pain. It was dated 1985, when, in her mind, her life had ended due to the accident.

Melinda and her husband had six wonderful, talented daughters and several grandchildren. Gradually, through mindfulness and learning to live in the moment, a consultation that identified some needed changes in medication, and two key consultations with other specialists, Melinda began to improve and take ownership of her life back.

Today she is still on medication and she meditates every day. Her favorite is the body scan. Recently, she has been able to travel a few times a year, including one trip on her own to the U.S. to stay with her daughters. She even went on shopping trips with them. Her husband often wipes tears from his eyes as he looks at her in our follow-up consultations. He is so proud of her and so grateful for the second chance at a happier life.

illness, pain, and biography

Certainly, there are times when an accident, injury or illness might come out of the blue, however ideal your life has been. But these adverse health events usually have a biography attached. You may be in the wrong place at the wrong time and someone drunk behind the wheel of a vehicle caused the accident that injured you, but then the biography that led to that event is the other driver's. Why was he/she drunk? What events had happened to him/her to cause him/her to choose to get drunk—and then drive—which then affected you? And let's hope your biography was a better one, one that allowed your stress systems to function well enough to permit you to recover completely from your injuries.

Certain diseases, such as severe acute respiratory syndrome (SARS) are very infectious, and just being in contact with a sufferer is all it takes to catch the disease. But those highly contagious and dangerous infections, which would likely infect you whether you have a healthy lifestyle or not, are rare. Your susceptibility to the majority of infectious diseases often *does* depend on your pre-existing life challenges and your lifestyle, which influence your resilience. Inadequate sleep, returning from a journey with jet lag, and being exposed to the cold in inadequate clothing are all examples of stressors that weaken your immune system and make it more likely you'll catch an infection if exposed.

Also, there are some diseases we inherit and suffer from if they are present in our genetic material, irrespective of stressors enabling them to be expressed: we have the disease if it is there and we don't if it isn't. Genetic diseases such as hemophilia or sickle-cell anemia are always expressed as the illness, but your caregivers will influence how well you deal with such illnesses. We have heard a hemophiliac's brother report that his brother had more bleeding into his joints when he was stressed. The vast majority of other diseases, however, such as diabetes and depression may manifest only if the stressors encountered during your life conspire to cause those genes to be expressed.

So since practicing mindfulness, it has become a "given" for us to look for events in our patients' lives to explain why their bodies malfunction when they do: these inquiries are made much more commonly in our psychiatric departments than in other clinics in our health care systems. We hope that changes, but our colleagues might comment that it would take more time to do their consultations, and they might not be sure how to change what they offer as solutions, even if they knew the triggering events.

Forty-year-old Robert, who came to the clinic using a cane to get help for his severe low-back pain, gave a tragic history of having injured his back in a bad fall at the age of eighteen, which led to his having to repeat a year in college after several months of being unable to move from his bed. Over the next few years, while still suffering from pain but managing it with medication and a good chiropractor, he built a career with a big company. But as the company expanded and their demands on him increased, his pain exacerbations became more frequent and eventually he left work and went on long-term disability.

Yet the MRI findings of his back showed nothing out of the ordinary. Some other medical history he related did suggest that he might have a disorder of his connective tissue: he had such severe reflux of stomach acid into his esophagus, he'd had to have surgery for it. But what we found interesting was that no one had ever asked him what was happening in his personal life when he was having these disabling episodes of back pain or esophageal reflux.

This man had coped with no less than seven episodes of his wife becoming manic. She'd had episodes when she made threats to his life, ran up huge bills on their credit cards, and was completely unable to care for their toddler son. Her first episode of mania had occurred within three years of their marriage and just after they had taken out a mortgage based on both of their incomes. And her income had then disappeared.

He had tried desperately to keep his job, flying all over the country, coping with jet lag, taking on too physical a role because he couldn't afford to be without the job, working through night shifts, and fielding calls from anxious family members and his wife when she was going into a manic episode. He was in Calgary when the police handcuffed her in Toronto and took her yet again into the ER for another assessment. She spent months in the hospital only to be discharged and then refuse to take her medications again.

Our mindfulness courses became a godsend for him: they became a huge piece of his pain management. He became aware of the triggers for his pain exacerbations, to see them clearly, and to manage them. When his wife was in a well phase, he brought her to our course. Two years later, she has remained stable and has not had another hospital admission.

the role of medication

This book was written *because* pain medications have not met their goal of reducing pain intensities for many of those disabled with severe long-term pain conditions, for long enough periods of time or with sufficiently tolerable side effects to return them to their original lives. Certainly, there is a place for using medications to decrease your pain enough to allow you to access the path to improvement: to tolerate more activity so you can strengthen your muscles to support your painful joints or back more effectively; to sleep better at night; or even to attend courses like our mindfulness classes, and be able to stay for the whole class. Skillfully used, medications can provide help for the transition.

Some people may need to stay on their medications for the long-term, when going without them entirely would be too painful. Some find that constant dosing with their meds does help them lead more productive lives and to continue working. For a more complete discussion of the medications for pain, you can go to www.painspeaking.com.

The Opioids

We have really strong pain medications available, morphine and related drugs, and even stronger opioids (narcotics), including hydromorphone (Dilaudid), fentanyl transdermal (Duragesic) (in patch form to go through the skin), oxycodone (OxyContin), hydrocodone (semi-synthetic opioid derived from two of the naturally occurring opiates: codeine and thebain), methadone (Dolophine, Amidone, and many others), diamorphine (heroin) and others, depending on the country in which you live. Ultram (tramadol hydrochloride), a weaker opioid, is also available in many parts of the world.

But even when the strong opiates work well for an individual, they often don't continue working that well for long. Doses have to be increased, and usually they don't take the pain away completely. They just reduce it—sometimes only for a while.

Moreover, when these drugs are stopped too suddenly, the withdrawal effects are most unpleasant. Drs. Jane Ballantyne and Jianren Mao of Massachusetts General Hospital Medical School, in their 2003 review of opioid therapy for chronic pain, describe many of the potential downsides for some of those on opioids. These include constipation, acid reflux, insomnia (opioids can interfere with restorative sleep), reduced oxygenation at night (sleep apnea), reduced effectiveness of the immune system, changed balances between hormones (loss of periods in women; low testosterone and sex drive in men), fluid retention in limbs, constant sleepiness without being able to sleep, lack of energy, and so on. Sometimes these side effects outweigh their benefits. Consequently, you may want to stop using opioids, by tapering off slowly, or reducing your dose under medical supervision.

Over time, you might begin to feel that your medication no longer works as well as when you first started it, and you may wonder whether the pain you feel now would be the same if you were to gradually discontinue using medication. After all, the painkillers may well be suppressing your own internal painkillers, your endorphins. And your clever body's systems have become more efficient at breaking down the drugs and flushing them out of your body, which is partly why they work less effectively now.

Note that if you miss a dose and observe the pain returning, that isn't good enough evidence that the meds still work: withdrawal from the drug during a missed dose manufactures *artificial* pain. In fact, large opioid doses, by mechanisms that may include suppressing your internal endorphins, can result in a tendency to feel *more* pain than usual, and not only as the dose wears off (Mao 2002).

Apparently, even your threshold to what you consider a painful stimulus can be reduced by being on long-term opioids: you may feel *any* pain more intensely. In the case of marihuana as a painkiller, for example, Dr. Mark Wallace and colleagues at the University of California (2007) demonstrated in an experiment that pot smokers who'd had a painful chili-pepper extract injected under their skin felt less pain only by smoking a moderate amount of marihuana. At higher doses, they felt *more* pain. This suggests that their internal natural painkillers are suppressed.

Nonopioids for Pain

Many of the drugs used to promote sleep (diazapam-related sedatives (Valium), amitriptyline-related sedative antidepressants); to reduce nerve irritation (anticonvulsants (gabapentin, pregabalin), tricyclic antidepressants (amitriptyline); as antidepressants or sedatives for the anxiety or depression that frequently accompanies pain conditions (paroxitene, imipramine); or as mild painkillers (nonsteroidal anti-inflammatories and acetaminophen) can interfere with other important body functions in addition to addressing the problems they are prescribed for. These other functions include: decreasing the amount of the deeper-sleep stages, impairing dental hygiene due to dry mouth, interfering with sexual function, affecting bowel, liver, kidney, bladder, blood pressure, cardiac functions and other systems, and affecting memory.

However, you may find just the right balance with the help of your health care professional, such that your pain decreases sufficiently to allow you to be more functional, and the side effects are minimal. In such circumstances, the pain might have been more stressful and destructive than the drugs are. That would tend to be more likely when the person is on the lower doses.

We may sound as if we deplore the medication interventions. We don't. We are glad we had a triptan (Imitrex, Zomig, Maxalt) available to take away migraines (Dr. Jackie) and the anticonvulsant (gabapentin, pregabalin) which managed the neuropathic leg pain after a surgical mishap (Lucie Costin-Hall). But when suffering from migraine and taking the triptan, an inventory takes place. Questions are asked: "Why is life out of balance enough to cause the migraine right now? Can I learn from this occasion and modify how much I cram into my life?"

a different way: aikido exercises revisited

You may wish to revisit chapter 9, People Stress, and this time replace the "attacker" in each of the four scenarios of the aikido exercises with your *pain*, whether it's physical or emotional. Are you aware of what your habit is in relating to your pain? Sitting with awareness of how you relate to your pain may result in reframing it, finding "the middle way," which is described in aikido exercise 4. As that unfolds, suffering lessens.

John

I used to get angry when my back pain started. If I had to mow the lawn I'd keep on going right through the pain getting worse. Talk about being "bent out of shape!" Now I pace myself, and I don't mind. I stop for a while just as the pain starts to increase, and I let it die down as I rest up and take in what's going on around me. I even notice sooner when I need to stop because I'm more mindful. I seem to know better how to move without making the pain get so bad, because I'm paying attention and treating my body better. The pain and me, well, we just have to get along together as best we can. And the strange thing is, I can do more now than I used to when I got angry and frustrated. Yes it takes longer. But the task still gets done.

A Journey with Pain

I decided to go for a drive
And, of course, my pain had to come with me.
I was just going out on a spring day
To see the country,
But pain came too.
My pain is fiery pain, a smoldering pain,
Who just stays with me.
So, I got in the car
And pain joined me in the front seat.
Sitting beside me, seat belt undone,
Defiant as always.
As I drove along, the pain grew
A nice inferno beside me.
I got to a rest stop I liked to frequent.
I got out of the car,
Stretched and sighed.
Breathing deeply, I moved my limbs,
And loosened my joints.
Pain grumpily exited the car,
Somewhat diminished
By my mindful movements.
I leaned on a picnic table
And drank in the scene
Fresh leaves on trees,
Wildflowers springing up from the ground,
The warm sun on my face,
The smell of a recent rain
I took the time,
Just for me.

Breathing deeply and soaking in
Each precious moment,
Moment by moment.
When I opened my eyes
I saw a flit of a bird.
I reached for my binoculars
And put them to my face.
The binoculars were backwards.
What was supposed to be big and close,
Was now small and far.
I was looking at a tree—a great distance away.
I laughed and swung around
To focus on my pain.
It was tiny and further away than ever before.
I lowered the glasses
And looked at the pain.
Straight on.
It really was small, but literally fuming.
I reached for my water bottle
And ever so carefully,
Dripped water all over what was left of the pain.
It spat and smoked and lost its power.
My pain was no more.
I smiled as I walked back to the car,
Got behind the wheel
And headed out
On a journey of my own.
Mindful to welcome
Each coming moment.

—Judy Gorman
Autumn, 2005

Most of all, be present for every lesson your body has to teach you. Be present for the challenges and be present for the consequences, in order to learn from them. Remember, it has not been the challenges themselves which caused the health/pain problems you have had, but the sheer intensity with which your mind reacted to them; that intensity was programmed by genetics and how you were nurtured during your formative years. That had consequences for your body: Inseparable from your mind.

Be present for the good times. Enjoy them. Know that the one certainty is that, moment to moment—your life/moods/emotions/body functions/pain—will all change. Look after your body and your mind: they're all you've got, and each affects the other constantly.

If you do the work in this book and stay with your mindfulness practice, your life *will* change. Your relationship with your pain *will* change—for the better. Be present for your life. Mindfully, with pain, or with less of it.

Perhaps, in time, your body *will* heal, but your mind likely has to heal first. And maybe one day the majority of your precious moments will be free of suffering.

> We must let go of the life we have planned, so as to accept the one that is waiting for us.
>
> —Joseph Campbell,
> From *Grief: The Silenced Emotion*

appendix

As stated in the introduction, the following tests could be done before you read and do the work in this book if you choose to. But they should certainly be repeated and compared when you finish reading and working with the book. If you keep up your practice over a few years, then they should be taken every six months after you complete your work with the book.

pain catastrophizing scale[*]

Date: _____

Everyone experiences painful situations at some point in their lives. Such experiences may include headaches, tooth pain, and joint or muscle pain. People are often exposed to situations that may cause pain, such as illness, injury, dental procedures or surgery.

You may be interested in the types of thoughts and feelings that you have when you are in pain. Listed below are thirteen statements describing different thoughts and feelings that may be associated with pain. Using the following scale, please indicate the degree to which you have these thoughts and feelings when you are experiencing pain.

0 = not at all
1 = to a slight degree
2 = to a moderate degree
3 = to a great degree
4 = all the time

[*]   Devised and tested by Michael Sullivan, Ph.D., 1995

When I'm in pain...

1. _____ I worry all the time about whether the pain will end.

2. _____ I feel I can't go on.

3. _____ It's terrible and I think it's never going to end.

4. _____ It's awful and I feel that it overwhelms me.

5. _____ I feel I can't stand it anymore.

6. _____ I become afraid that the pain will get worse.

7. _____ I keep thinking of other painful events.

8. _____ I anxiously want the pain to go away.

9. _____ I can't seem to keep it out of my mind.

10. _____ I keep thinking about how much it hurts.

11. _____ I keep thinking about how badly I want the pain to stop.

12. _____ There's nothing I can do to reduce the intensity of the pain.

13. _____ I wonder whether something serious may happen.

_____ *Total*

Adding the scores: The maximum you can score is 52. The average for the Canadian pain population before they take our course is around 30. It drops to an average of about 24 after one course. The normal U.S. population average is around 17. Adding the scores to questions 6, 7, and 13 will provide you with a measure of how much you magnify your pain. Questions 8, 9, 10, and 11 added together will tell you how much you ruminate on pain, and adding the scores of questions 1, 2, 3, 4, 5 and 12 will give you a measure of how helpless you feel. Doing this test after you finish reading the book, and every six months after that, for some time will show you what is happening to your pain catastrophizing thinking, which is related to how disabled you are.

numeric pain scale[**]

On a scale of 0 to 10, where 0 represents no pain and 10 represents excruciating pain, please circle the number which best represents your pain level:

Right now:

0   1   2   3   4   5   6   7   8   9   10

At its best during the past week:

0   1   2   3   4   5   6   7   8   9   10

At its worst during the past week:

0   1   2   3   4   5   6   7   8   9   10

As it is usually:

0   1   2   3   4   5   6   7   8   9   10

[**]   Farrar et al. 2001

modified PRISM (pictorial representation of illness and self measure) test (to monitor suffering)***

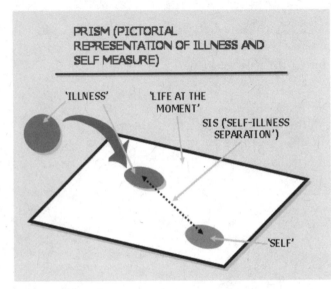

PRISM (PICTORIAL
REPRESENTATION OF ILLNESS AND
SELF MEASURE)

'ILLNESS' 'LIFE AT THE
MOMENT'

SIS ('SELF-ILLNESS
SEPARATION')

'SELF'

Use a letter sized (8.5" x 11") piece of paper to represent your life, and draw a 2 ¾" diameter circle in the lower right-hand corner as illustrated: this represents your concept of self. Then draw approximately 2" diameter circles to represent the other factors in your life: pain (disease), family, partner, work, and recreation. Draw the pain disc first, whether you suffer from emotional or physical pain, positioning it in relation to your "self" disc to represent its intrusiveness into your life. Then draw in the other discs, where applicable, to represent their importance or place in your life. Over time these positions may change, and you may find it thought-provoking to do this and see the changes. When we measure the distance between the centers of these discs at several times during the patient's life, it becomes a quantitative way of representing and recording what is happening. This PRISM test is thought to be a way to measure suffering.

*** Büchi et al. 1998

recommended reading

Bested, A., A. C. Logan, and R. Howe. 2006. *Chronic Fatigue Syndrome and Fibromyalgia*. Tennessee: Cumberland House.

Brantley, J. 2003. *Calming Your Anxious Mind*. Oakland, CA: New Harbinger Publications Inc.

Dahl, J., and T. Lundgren. 2006. *Living Beyond Your Pain*. Oakland, CA: New Harbinger Publications Inc.

Doidge, N. 2007. *The Brain That Changes Itself*. New York: Viking.

Eifert, G. H., M. McKay, J. P. Forsyth. 2006. *ACT on Life, Not on Anger*. Oakland, CA: New Harbinger Publications Inc.

Fischgrund S., A., and R. Hiatt-Coblentz. 2006. *Pilates for Fragile Backs*. Oakland, CA: New Harbinger Publications Inc.

Gardner-Nix, J., and L. Costin Hall. 2004. *Painspeaking: A Pain Clinic in a Box*. Pathfinder communications: Toronto. Available online at www.painspeaking.com. 4 compact disc set.

Goleman, D. 2003. *Destructive Emotions*. New York: Bantam Dell.

———. 1995. *Emotional Intelligence*. New York: Bantam Books.

Hayes, S. C., and S. Smith. 2005. *Get Out of Your Mind & Into Your Life*. Oakland, CA: New Harbinger Publications Inc.

Kabat-Zinn. J. 2005. *Coming to Our Senses*. New York: Hyperion.

———. 1994. *Wherever You Go There You Are*. New York: Hyperion.

Lipton, B. 2005. *The Biology of Belief: Unleashing the Power of Consciousness, Matter and Miracles*. Santa Rosa, CA: Mountain of Love/Elite Books.

Mason, P. T. and R. Kreger. 1998. *Stop Walking on Eggshells*. Oakland, CA: New Harbinger Publications Inc.

Rothschild, B. 2000. *The Body Remembers: The Psychophysiology of Trauma and Trauma Treatment*. W. W. New York: Norton & Company.

Santorelli, S. 1999. *Heal Thyself*. New York: Bell Tower.

Schneider, J. 2004. *Living with Chronic Pain*. Healthy New York: Living Books.

Seligman, M. E. P. 2002. *Authentic Happiness*. New York: The Free Press.

Siegal, B. 1989. *Peace, Love and Healing*. New York: Harper Perennial.

———. 1986. *Love, Medicine, and Miracles*. New York: Harper and Row.

Siegal, D. J. 2007. *The Mindful Brain: Reflection and Attunement in the Cultivation of Well-Being*. New York: W. W. Norton & Company.

Tolle, E. 1999. *Practicing the Power of Now*. 1999. Novato, CA: New World Library.

Weil, A., and J. Kabat-Zinn. 2005. *Meditation for Optimum Health: How to use mindfulness and breathing to heal your body and refresh your mind*. Louisville, CO: Sounds True.

references

Amanzio, M., and F. Benedetti. 1999. Neuropharmacological dissection of placebo analgesia: Expectation-activated opioid systems versus conditioning-activated specific subsystems. *Journal of Neuroscience* 19: 484-494.

Andrews, V. H., and H. R. Hall. 1990. The effects of relaxation/imagery training on recurrent aphthous stomatitis: A preliminary study. *Psychosomatic Medicine* 52 (5): 526-535.

Arnsten P., and S. Goldman-Rakic. 1998. Noise stress impairs prefrontal cortical cognitive function in monkeys: Evidence for a hyperdopaminergic mechanism. *Archives of General Psychology* 55: 362-368.

Aron, E. N. 1996. *The Highly Sensitive Person: How to Thrive When the World Overwhelms You.* New York: Broadway Books.

Ballantyne, J. C., and J. Mao. 2003. Opioid therapy for chronic pain. *New England Journal of Medicine* 349: 1943-1953.

Benedetti, F. 2007. What do you expect from this treatment? *Pain* 128: 193-194.

Benedetti, F., A. Pollo, G. Maggi, S., Vighetti, and I. Rainero. 2002. Placebo analgesia: From physiological mechanisms to clinical implications. Proceedings of the 10th World Congress on Pain, edited by J. Dostrovsky, D. B. Carr, and M. Koltzenburg. *Progress in Pain Research and Management* 24: 315-323. IASP Press. Seattle, WA.

Block, G., B. Patterson, and A. Subar. 1992. Fruit, vegetables, and cancer prevention: A review of the epidemiological evidence. *Nutrition and Cancer* 18 (1): 1-29.

Boden S., D. Davis, T. Dina, N. Patronas, and S. Wiesel. 1990. Abnormal magnetic resonance scans of the lumbar spine in asymptomatic subjects. *Journal of Bone Joint Surgery* 72: 403-408.

Boos, N., R. Reider, V. Schade, K. Spratt, N. Semmer, and M. Aebi. 1995. The diagnostic accuracy of magnetic resonance imaging, work perception and psychosocial factors in identifying symptomatic disc herniation. *Spine* 20: 2613-2625.

Braly, J., and R. Hoggan. 2002. *Dangerous Grains.* New York: Avery.

Breen, C., A. Crowe, H. J. Roelfsema, I. Singh Saluja, D. Guenter, J. Schoenen, et al. 1998. Effectiveness of high-dose riboflavin in migraine prophylaxis: A randomized controlled trial. *Neurology* 50: 466-470.

Brizendine, L. 2006. *The Female Brain.* New York: Broadway Books.

Bruehl S., J. W. Burns, O. Y. Chung, B. Johnson, and P. Ward. 2002. Anger and pain sensitivity in chronic low-back pain patients and pain-free controls: The role of endogenous opioids. *Pain* 99 (1-2): 223-233.

Bruehl S., O. Y. Chung, J. W. Burns, and S. Biridepalli. 2003. The association between anger expression and chronic pain intensity: Evidence for partial mediation by endogenous opioid dysfunction. *Pain* 106 (3): 317-324.

Büchi, S., T. Sensky, L. Sharpe, and N. Timberlake. 1998. Graphic representation of illness: A novel method of measuring patients' perceptions of the impact of illness. *Psychotherapy & Psychosomatic Medicine.* 67 (4-5): 222-225.

Caples, S. M., A. S. Gami, K. Virend, and V. K. Somers. 2005. Obstructive sleep apnea. *Annals of Internal Medicine* 142: 187-197.

Carson J. W., F. J. Keefe, V. Goli, A. M. Fras, T. R. Lynch, S. R. Thorp, et al. 2005. Forgiveness and chronic low-back pain: A preliminary study examining the relationship of forgiveness to pain, anger, and psychological distress. *Pain* 6: 84-91.

Cohen, S., M. Cuneyt, M. D. Alper, W. J. Doyle, J. J. Treanor, and R. B. Turner. 2006. Positive emotional style predicts resistance to illness after experimental exposure to rhinovirus or influenza virus. *Psychosomatic Medicine* 68: 809-815.

Darling, M. 1991. The use of exercise as a method of aborting migraine. *Headache: Journal of Head & Face Pain.* 31 (9): 616-618.

Davidson, R. J., J. Kabat-Zinn, J. Schumacher, M. Rosenkranz, D. Muller, S. F. Santorelli, et al. 2003. Alterations in brain and immune function produced by mindfulness meditation. *Psychotherapy and Psychosomatic Medicine* 65: 564-570.

DeCharms, R. C., F. Maeda, G. H. Glover, D. Ludlow, J. M. Pauly, D. Soneji, et al. 2005. Control over brain activation and pain learned by using real-time functional MRI. *Proceedings of the National Academy of Sciences* 102 (51): 18626–18631.

Farrar, J. T., J. P. Young, L. LaMoreaux, J. L. Werth, and R. M. Poole. 2001. Clinical importance of changes in chronic pain intensity measured on an 11-point numeric pain rating scale. *Pain* 94: 149-158.

Gilbert, E. 2006. *Eat, Pray, Love.* New York: Penguin Books.

Goldstein, L. E., A. M. Rasmusson, B. Steve Bunney, and R. H. Roth. 1996. Role of the amygdala in the coordination of behavioral, neuroendocrine, and prefrontal cortical monoamine responses to psychological stress in the rat. *Journal of Neuroscience* 16 (15): 4787-4798.

Goleman, D. J., and G. E. Schwartz. 1979. Meditation as an intervention in stress reactivity. *Journal of Consulting and Clinical Psychology* 44 (3): 456-466.

Grzesiak, R. C. 2003. Revisiting pain-prone personalities: Combining psychodynamics with the neurobiological sequelae of trauma. *American Journal of Pain Management* 13: 6-15.

Guess, H. A., A. Kleinman, J. W. Kusek, and L. W. Engel, eds. 2002. *The Science of the Placebo: Toward an Interdisciplinary Research Agenda.* London: Medical Journal Books.

Heffner, K. L., J. K. Kiecolt-Glaser, T. J. Loving, R. Glaser, and W. B. Malarkey. 2004. Spousal support satisfaction as a modifier of physiological responses to marital conflict in younger and older couples. *Journal of Behavioral Medicine* 27 (3): 233-254.

Heim, C., D. J. Newport, S. Heit, Y. P. Graham, M. Wilcox, R. Bonsall, et al. 2000. Increased pituitary-adrenal and autonomic responses to stress in adult women after sexual and physical abuse in childhood. *JAMA* 284 (5): 592-597.

Hellhammer, D. 2006. Baby girls born to mothers burdened by stress may be at risk for fibromyalgia. Paper presented at International Congress of Neuroendocrinology June 19–22, 2006. Pittsburgh, PA.

Hoffman, B. M., R. K. Papas, D. K. Chatkoff, and R. D. Kerns. 2007. Meta-analysis of psychological intervention for chronic low back pain. *Health Psychology* 26 (1): 1-9.

Hohmann, A. G., R. L. Suplita, N. M. Bolton, M. H. Neely, D. Fegley, R. Mangieri, et al. 2005. An endocannabinoid mechanism for stress-induced analgesia. *Nature* 435 (7045): 1108-1112.

Hooten, M. W., M. K. Turner, and J. E. Schmidt. 2007. Prevalence and clinical correlates of vitamin D inadequacy among patients with chronic pain. *Anesthesiology* 107: A1380.

Jackson, T., T. Iezza, H. Chen, S. Ebnet, and K. Eglitis. 2005. Gender, interpersonal transactions, and the perception of pain: An experimental analysis. *Journal of Pain* 6: 228-236.

Kabat-Zinn, J., E. Wheeler, T. Light, A. Skillings, M. S. Scharf, T. G. Cropley, et al. 1998. Influence of a mindfulness-based stress reduction intervention on rates of skin clearing in patients with moderate to severe psoriasis undergoing phototherapy (UVB) and photochemotherapy (PUVA). *Psychotherapy and Psychosomatic Medicine* 60: 625-632.

Kabat-Zinn, J. 1991. *Full Catastrophe Living: Using the Wisdom of Your Body and Mind to Face Stress, Pain, and Illness.* New York: Dell Paperback.

Kiecolt-Glaser, J. K., K. J. Preacher, R. C. MacCallum, C. Atkinson, W. B. Malarkey, and R. Glaser. 2003. Chronic stress and age-related increases in the proinflammatory cytokine IL-6. *Proceedings of the National Academy of Science* 100 (15): 9090-9095.

Kiecolt-Glaser, J. K., G. C. Page, P. T. Marucha, R. C. MacCallum, and R. Glaser. 1998. Psychological influences on surgical recovery: Perspectives from psychoneuroimmunology. *American Psychologist* 55: 1209-1218.

Kiecolt-Glaser, J. K., J. R Dura, C. E. Speicher, O. J. Trask, and R. Glaser. 1991. Spousal caregivers of dementia victims: Longitudinal changes in immunity and health. *Psychosomatic Medicine* 53: 345-362.

Knight J. A. 2000. Free radicals, antioxidants and the immune system. *Annals of Clinical and Laboratory Science Review* 30 (2): 145-158.

Koseoglu, E., A. Akboyraz, A. Soyuer, and A. O. Ersoy AO. 2003. Aerobic exercise and plasma beta endorphin levels in patients with migrainous headache without aura. *Cephalalgia* 23 (10): 972-976.

Lavigne, G., B. Sessle, M. Choiniere, and P. J. Soja. 2007. *Sleep and Pain.* Seattle: IASP Press.

Levine, J. D., and N. C. Gordon. 1984. Influence of the method of drug administration on analgesic response. *Nature* 312: 755-756.

Liddle, S. D., G. D. Baxter, and J. H. Gracey. 2004. Exercise and chronic low-back pain: What works? *Pain* 107: 176-190.

Linde, K., C. M. Witt, A. Streng, W. Weidenhammer, S. Wagenpfeil, B. Brinkhaus, S. N. Willich, and D. Melchart. 2007. The impact of patient expectations on outcomes in four randomized controlled trials of acupuncture in patients with chronic pain. *Pain* 128 (3): 264-71.

Mao, J. 2002. Opioid-induced abnormal pain sensitivity: Implications in clinical opioid therapy. *Pain* 100: 213-217.

Mayo Clinic. 2005. Meditation: Focusing your mind to achieve stress reduction. April. www.mayoclinic.com/health/meditation/HQ01070. Accessed May 2, 2008.

McBeth, J., Y. H. Chiu, A. J. Silman, D. Ray, R. Morriss, C. Dickens, et al. 2005. Hypothalamic-pituitary-adrenal stress axis function and the relationship with chronic widespread pain and its antecedents. *Arthritis Research and Therapy* 5: R992-R1000.

McCracken L. M., and C. Eccleston. 2005. A prospective study of acceptance of pain and patient functioning with chronic pain. *Pain* 118: 164-169.

McEwen, B. S., C. Liston, and J. H. Morrison. 2006. Stress-induced structural plasticity in prefrontal cortex, amygdala and hippocampus. *Neuropsychopharmacology.* S13 (Dec. 31).

McEwen, B. S., and E. N. Lasley. 2002. *The End of Stress as We Know It.* Washington, D.C.: Dana Press.

Meaney, M. J., and M. Szyf. 2005. Maternal care as a model for experience-dependent chromatin plasticity? *Trends in Neuroscience* 28 (9): 456-463.

Miller-Butterworth, C. M., J. R. Kaplan, J. Shaffer, B. Devlin, S. B. Manuck, and R. E. Ferrell. 2008. Sequence variation in the primate dopamine transporter gene and its relationship to social dominance. *Molecular Biology and Evolution.* 25 (1): 18-28.

Moody, L. E., M. Fraser, and H. Yarandi. 1993. Effects of guided imagery in patients with chronic bronchitis and emphysema. *Clinical Nursing Research* 2 (4): 478-486.

Moulin, D., A. J. Clark, M. Speechley, and P. K. Morley-Forster. 2002. Chronic pain in Canada: Prevalence, treatment, impact and role of opioid analgesia. *Pain Research and Management* 7 (4): 170-173.

Naperstek, B. 1994. *Staying Well with Guided Imagery: How to Harness the Power of Your Imagination for Health and Healing.* New York: Warner Books.

Pasternak, G. W. 2001. The pharmacology of mu analgesics: From patients to genes. *Neuroscientist* 7: 220-231.

Pert, C. B. 1997. *Molecules of Emotion: Why You Feel the Way You Feel.* New York: Scribners.

Real, Terrence. 1997. *I Don't Want To Talk About It.* New York: Scribners.

Reed, Barbara. 1983. *Food, Teens and Behavior.* Manitowoc, WI: Natural Press.

Rosengren, S., S. Hawken, K. Ôunpuu, M. Sliwa, W. Zubaid, K. Almahmeed, et al. 2004. Association of psychosocial risk factors with risk of acute myocardial infarction in 11,119 cases and 13,648 controls from 52 countries (the INTERHEART study): Case control study. *The Lancet* 364 (9438): 953-962.

Sarno, J. 1998. *The Mindbody Prescription: Healing the Body, Healing the Pain.* New York: Warner Books.

Schofferman, J., D. Anderson, R. Hines, G. Smith, and G. Keane. 1993. Childhood psychological trauma and chronic refractory low-back pain. *Clinical Journal of Pain* 4: 260-265.

Seligman, M. E. P. 1990. *Learned Optimism.* New York: Pocket Books.

Spradlin, S. E. 2002. *Don't Let Your Emotions Run Your Life: How Dialectical Behavior Therapy Can Put You in Control.* Oakland, CA: New Harbinger Publications.

Sullivan, M. J., S. R. Bishop, and J. Pivik. 1995. The pain catastrophizing scale: Development and validation. *Psychological Assessment* 7 (4): 524-532.

Takamatsu, H., A. Noda, Y. Murakami, M. Tatsumi, R. Ichise, S. Nishimura, et al. 2003. A PET study following treatment with a pharmacological stressor, FG7142, in conscious monkeys. *Brain Research* 980: 275-280.

Turk, D. C., and R. Gatchel. 2002. *Psychological Approaches to Pain Management: A Practitioner's Handbook,* 2nd ed. New York: Guilford Press.

Villemure C., S. Wassimi, G. J. Bennett, Y. Shir, and M. C. Bushnell. 2006. Unpleasant odors increase pain processing in a patient with neuropathic pain: Psychophysical and fMRI investigation. *Pain* 120: 213-220.

Villemure, C., B. M. Slotnick, and M. C. Bushnell. 2003. Dissociation of attentional and emotional modulation of pain using pleasant and unpleasant odors in humans. *Pain* 106: 101-108.

Wada, M., C. DeLong, C. J. Hong, Y. H. Rieke, and I. Song. 2007. Enzymes and receptors of prostaglandin pathways with arachidonic acid-derived versus eicosapentaenoic acid-derived substrates and products. *Journal of Biological Chemistry* 282: 22254-22266.

Wallace, M., G. Schulteis, J. H. Atkinson, T. Wolfson, D. Lazzaretto, H. Bentley, et al. 2007. Dose-dependent effects of smoked cannabis on capsaicin-induced pain and hyperalgesia in healthy volunteers. *Anesthesia* 107 (5): 785-796.

Welberg, L. A. M., and J. R. Seckl. 2001. Prenatal stress, glucocorticoids and the programming of the brain. *Journal of Neuroendocrinology* 13: 113-128.

Wood, P. B. 2004. Stress and dopamine: Implications for the pathophysiology of chronic widespread pain. *Medical Hypotheses* 62 (3): 420-424.

Zachariae, R. J. S., P. Kristensen, J. Hokland, E. Ellegaard, E. Metze, and M. Hokland. 1990. Effect of psychological intervention in the form of relaxation and guided imagery on cellular immune function in normal healthy subjects: An overview. *Journal of Psychotherapy & Psychosomatic Medicine* 54 (1): 32-39.

Zubieta, J-K., Y. R. Smith, J. A. Bueller, Y. Xu, M. R. Kilbourn, D. M. Jewett, et al. 2001. Regional mu opioid receptor regulation of sensory and affective dimensions of pain. *Science* 293: 311-315.

Zubieta, J-K, M. M. Heitzeg, Y. R Smith, J. A. Bueller, K. Xu, Y. Xu, R. A. Koeppe, C. S. Stohler, and D. Goldman. 2003. COMT genotype affects neurotransmitter responses to a pain stressor. *Science* 299: 1240-1243.

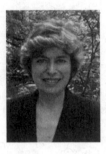 **Dr. Jackie Gardner-Nix** is a physician and chronic pain consultant at St. Michael's Hospital and the Sunnybrook Health Sciences Centre in Toronto, Canada. She is assistant professor in the department of anesthesia at the University of Toronto. Gardner-Nix has been on advisory boards for the Ontario College of Physicians and Surgeons, the Ontario Medical Association, the Ontario Ministry of Health, and a number of pharmaceutical companies. She is an accomplished speaker who has given many workshops and presentations internationally and has written publications on control of chronic non-cancer pain and on palliative care. Gardner-Nix was a Toronto Sun "Women on the Move" nominee in 1994 for her work in pain and symptom control.

Lucie Costin-Hall, MA, currently works with Jackie Gardner-Nix as a cofacilitator of mindfulness-based chronic pain management (MBCPM) workshops for patients at two teaching hospitals in Toronto and at numerous distant sites throughout Ontario via the interactive conferencing technology of the Ontario Telehealth Network (OTN). In the last five years, more than 2,000 chronic pain patients have participated in these workshops. Before discovering the mindfulness program, Costin-Hall was a chronic pain sufferer.

Jon Kabat-Zinn, Ph.D., is internationally known for his work as a scientist, writer, and meditation teacher engaged in bringing mindfulness into the mainstream of medicine and society. He is professor of medicine emeritus at the University of Massachusetts Medical School and author of numerous books, including *Full Catastrophe Living, Arriving at Your Own Door*, and *Coming to Our Senses*.

index

brain: female, 125-126; fight-or-flight response and, 60-62; higher centers of, 59; pain responses and, 57, 58
brain fog, 68
Braly, James, 109
break taking, 44-45
breathing, 32, 35
Brizendine, Louann, 125
bronchitis, 163
Bushnell, Catherine, 48, 75

C

caffeine, 112, 118
Cameron, Julia, 134
Campbell, Joseph, 189
canker sores, 163
cannabinoids, 65
CDs: body scan, 79; guided imagery, 165; guided meditation, 37, 40; movement meditation, 101
celiac disease, 108
children: art therapy with, 161; body memory and, 70-72; meditation and, 50-51; stress in, 64, 66
chocolate, 106
chronic fatigue syndrome (CFS), 157
chronic pain, 2. See also pain
chronic stress, 21
cleaning mindfully, 47
coffee, 112
Cohen, Sheldon, 62
cold pressor test, 124
computer use, 118
COMT gene, 20, 75
corticotrophin-releasing factor (CRF), 60
cortisol, 60, 63, 65-66, 68
courses in chronic pain management, 11

D

Dangerous Grains (Braly & Hoggan), 109
daytime naps, 119

defusion, 129
dehydration, 113
depression: genetics and, 20; REM sleep and, 116
dermatitis herpetiformis, 109
Descartes, René, 56-57
diabetes, 111
dialectical behavioral therapy (DBT), 129-130
dialectical thinking, 130-131
dichotomous thinking, 130
diet. See eating habits; food
directed concentration, 32
distraction, 48, 70
doctor visits, 177-179
Don't Let Your Emotions Run Your Life (Spradlin), 130
dopamine, 65
drugs. See medications

E

Eat, Pray, Love (Gilbert), 115
eating habits, 107-114; immune system and, 113; meal preparation and, 105-106; mindfulness and, 105-107; moods and behaviors and, 110-113; pain and, 107-110; sleep hygiene and, 118; vitamins and, 113-114; weight loss and, 106-107. See also food
emotions: artwork and, 134-135, 160; doctor visits and, 177-179; mindfulness and, 25-26; pain and, 5-7, 10, 12, 21-22, 76; relationships and, 126-129; stress and, 53; writing and, 156-159, 160. See also moods
emphysema, 163
End of Stress as We Know It, The (McEwen), 62
endogenous opioids, 71
endorphins, 57, 65, 71, 74-75, 115, 185
epigenetics, 22
exercise, 114-115, 118
explicit memory, 71

F

facial expressions, 125
failure, fear of, 30
"Farmer and His Horse" fable, 27-28
feelings. *See emotions*
Female Brain, The (Brizendine), 125
fibromyalgia: drawings inspired by, 144-147; exercise and, 115; sleep and, 67-68, 117; stress and, 65-66
fight-or-flight response, 19, 60-61
five-minute meditation, 35-36
flashbacks, 37, 54, 85
flinching response, 59
fluids, 113
food: allergies related to, 108; caffeine and, 112; calories in, 106; gluten sensitivity and, 108-109; glycemic index and, 111-112; immune system and, 113; lactose intolerance and, 110; migraines and, 107-108; moods and behaviors and, 110-113; pain and, 107-110; sleep and, 118; vitamins and, 113-114. *See also eating habits*
Food, Teens and Behavior (Reed), 110
formal meditation practice, 32
Full Catastrophe Living (Kabat-Zinn), 32, 115, 126, 157
functional MRIs (fMRIs), 48, 69-70, 75

G

Gandhi, Mohandas K., 121
Gatchel, Robert, 75
gender differences, 124-126; female brain and, 125-126; pain and, 124
genetics: diseases caused by, 182; epigenetics and, 22; life events and, 18-19; pain and, 7, 20
Gilbert, Elizabeth, 115
Glaser, Ronald, 62
gluten sensitivity, 108-109
glycemic index, 111-112
goals, 39

Gorman, Judy, 188
Guernica (Picasso), 134
guided imagery, 162-173; artwork and, 165; definition of, 162; example of using, 164; immune system and, 162-163; meditation using, 165-169; mindfulness and, 163. *See also visualization*
guided meditation CDs, 37, 40

H

Hatha yoga, 115
health: physical needs and, 103-104; stress and, 21, 62-63
helping others, 160
helplessness, 179-181
highly sensitive individuals, 19-20
Highly Sensitive Person: How to Thrive When the World Overwhelms You, The (Aron), 15, 19
Hines-Brown test, 124
hippocampus, 58, 70
Hippocrates, 103
Hiroto, Donald, 180
Hoggan, Ron, 109
Hohmann, Andrea, 65
Hooten, Michael, 114
hormones, 17; opioid medications and, 184; stress, 19, 45, 60-62, 64
hydrocephalus, 139
hyperalgesia, 65
hypothalamus-pituitary-adrenal (HPA) axis, 60-62; fight-or-flight response and, 60-61; immune system and, 61-62; neocortex and, 62

I

I Don't Want to Talk About It (Real), 21
illness, 182
"I'm Drowning in My Own Pain" (drawing), 151
imagery: cultural use of, 162. *See also guided imagery; visualization*

immune system: foods and, 113; guided imagery and, 162-163; infectious diseases and, 182; meditation and, 33; sleep and, 62, 104; stress and, 18, 19, 61-62
impatience, 85
implicit memory, 71, 72
infectious diseases, 182
informal meditation practice, 32
insulin, 111, 112
interpersonal interactions, 125
irritable bowel syndrome (IBS), 68, 109

JKL

journaling. *See writing*
"Journey with Pain, A" (Gorman), 187-188
judgments, 27, 42-43
Kabat-Zinn, Jon, v, 1, 8, 10, 19, 32, 55, 89, 115, 126, 157, 170, 171
Kaplan, Jay, 64
Kiecolt-Glaser, Janice, 62
lactose intolerance, 110
lake meditation, 170-171
Lancet, The (journal), 22
learned helplessness, 180
Learned Optimism (Seligman), 179
life trauma: pain and, 7. *See also traumatic memories*
limbic system, 58

M

Magnetic Resonance Images (MRIs), 5
Mao, Jianren, 184
marihuana, 185
martial arts exercises, 126-130
McBeth, John, 65
McEwen, Bruce S., 62-63
meal preparation, 105-106
Meaney, Michael, 64
measurement scales: Numeric Pain Scale, 193; Pain Catastrophizing Scale, 191-192
Medical Hypotheses (journal), 65

medications, 183-186; meditation and, 18, 33, 52; nonopioid, 185-186; opioid, 119, 184-185; pain treated with, 3-5; side effects of, 184, 185; sleep, 119
meditation, 31-41, 49-55; breathing and, 32, 35; CDs for guiding, 37; challenges of, 49-55; clothing for, 34; committing to daily, 54-55; definitions of, 31-32; discomfort during, 34-35; duration of, 34, 37, 40; emotional stress and, 53; falling asleep during, 51; five-minute, 35-36; flashbacks during, 54; guided imagery, 165-169; guidelines for, 39-40; kids and pets and, 50-51; medication and, 18, 33, 52; mental restlessness and, 49-50; mindfulness and, vii, 31; noisy environments and, 51-52; pain and, 34-35, 52; physical benefits of, 33; positions for, 34; relaxation vs., 32-33; starting to practice, 33-35; stress and, 55; timing of, 33, 50; visualization, 170-173; walking, 37
"Meditation for Optimal Health" CD (Weil), 32
memories: body-based, 70-72; traumatic, 54, 64, 66, 70-72
mental restlessness, 49-50
migraine headaches: exercise and, 114; food and, 107-108; stress and, 45
milk products, 110
mind-body connection, 13, 17-19; chemistry of thought and, 17-18; nature/nurture and, 18-19. *See also body; brain*
Mindbody Prescription: Healing the Body, Healing the Pain (Sarno), 9
mindfulness: acceptance and, 44; attitudes associated with, 26-30; authors' first experiences with, 8-10; break taking and, 44-45; cleaning with, 47; courses on pain

management using, 11; definition of, 23; distraction and, 48; eating with, 107-109; emotions and, 25-26; guided imagery and, 163; meditation and, vii, 31; reclaiming, 24-25; showering with, 46-47; vacations and, 24; visualization and, 163

mindfulness-based chronic pain management (MBCPM), ix, 11

mindfulness-based stress reduction (MBSR), vii

Molecules of Emotion (Pert), 56

monkey mind, 50

Montapert, Alfred A., 162

moods: expressing though artwork or writing, 160; food influencing behaviors and, 110-113. *See also emotions*

morphine, 184

mountain meditation, 171

movement meditation, 88-102; illustrated instructions for, 91-101; mentally preparing for, 89; orientation to, 89-90; pros and cons of, 88-89

"My Bed" (drawing), 150

"My Overall Mood" (drawing), 143

"My Pain" (drawing), 138

"My Pain" (poem), 158-159

"My Pain Experience" (drawing), 149

"My Pain Troll" (drawings), 152, 153

N

naloxone, 73

Naperstek, Belleruth, 169

naps, 119

narcotics, 3, 184-185

natural killer (NK) cells, 162-163

nature and nurture, 18-19

Nature (journal), 65

Nature of Things–Passion and Fury: Anger, The (Suzuki), 18

neocortex, 59, 62

neuropathic pain, 9, 116

neurotransmitters, 17

Nhat Hanh, Thich, 16, 42

noisy environments, 51-52

nonopioid medications, 185-186

nonstriving attitude, 39, 55

"not right" relationships, 132-133

Numeric Pain Scale, 193

OPQ

Oliver, Jaimie, 110

Omega-3 fatty acids, 113

opioid medications, 119, 184-185

optimism, 180

Oracle of Delphi, 77

pain: aikido exercises and, 186; anticipation of, 74; artificial, 185; artwork inspired by, 135-155; biography and, 181-182; eating habits and, 107-110; emotions and, 5-7, 10, 12, 21-22, 76; exercise and, 114-115; explanation of, 57; fluids and, 113; gender and, 124; genetics and, 7, 20; illness and, 182; intensification of, 84-85; life trauma and, 7, 71-72; medications for, 3-5, 183-186; meditation and, 34-35, 52; memory of, 69, 70-72; mental reduction of, 74-75; mindful understanding of, 12-13; placebo response and, 73-74; proving to others, 69-70; relationships and, 126-130; secondary gain and, 175-177; situations affecting, 43-44; sleep and, 117; stress and, 45, 65-66; vitamins and, 113-114; writings inspired by, 156-159

Pain Catastrophizing Scale, 181, 191-192

Pain Speaking CD, 165

painspeaking.com website, 37, 79, 101

palliative care, 3, 8

Parkinson's disease, 109

patience, 29-30

stress-induced analgesia, 64-65
subconscious secondary gain, 175-177
Sullivan, Michael, 181
superwoman high achiever, 20
Suzuki, David, 18

TUV

telemedicine courses, 11
tend and befriend strategy, 126
thalamus, 57
"This is the Pain that Surrounds My
    Life" (drawing), 155
thought: awareness of, 50; chemistry
    of, 17-19; dialectical, 130-131;
    dichotomous, 130; meditation and,
    40; pain reduction and, 74-75
"Tied Up in Knots" (drawing), 137
tone of voice, 129-130
traumatic memories: body-based,
    70-72; chronic stress and, 64, 66;
    meditation and, 54; pain and, 7
triggers, 108
trust, 29
TV watching, 118
vacations, 5-6, 24
Van Gogh, Vincent, 134
"Verbal Picture of My Migraine Pain"
    (essay), 156-157
visualization, 170-173; definition of,
    163; meditations using, 170-173;
    movement meditation and, 89. *See
    also guided imagery*
vitamins, 113-114
voice, tone of, 129-130

W

"Waiting Game, The" (drawing), 138
walking meditation, 37
Wallace, Mark, 185
weight loss, 106-107
Weil, Andrew, 32
Wood, Patrick, 65
writing, 156-161; acceptance through,
    161; examples from pain sufferers,
    156-159; expressing pain through,
    160

XYZ

"Year in the Life of My Pain, A"
    (drawings), 144, 145, 146
yoga, 115
Zubieta, Jon-Kar, 74

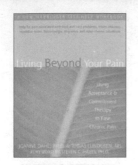
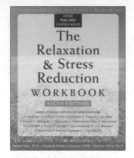
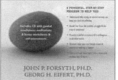
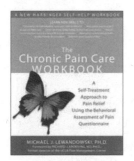
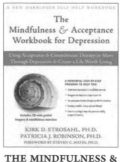
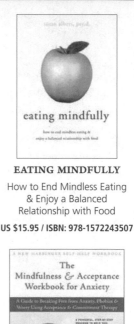